THE

KT DIET
28-DAY
MEAL PLAN

dR

IT TAKES
4 WEEKS
FOR YOU TO NOTICE A CHANGE.

IT TAKES
8 WEEKS
FOR YOUR FRIENDS TO NOTICE.

IT TAKES
12 WEEKS
FOR THE REST OF THE WORLD TO NOTICE.

IT TAKES
1 MOMENT
FOR YOU TO DECIDE YOU'RE WORTH IT.

KT
DIET
KETO FOR LIFE

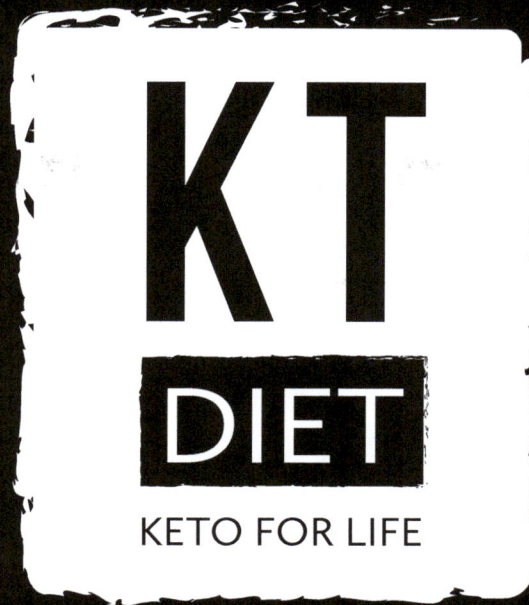

KETO TRANSFORMATION

THE **ULTIMATE KETO MEAL PLAN** TO GET YOU

FIT,

FOCUSED,

AND

FABULOUS.

DRAEKK

DRAEKK

NOTICE

This book is intended as a reference only, not as a medical manual. This book is not intended to be an exhaustive overview, but is designed to aid the reader to make informed decisions about health, diet, and exercise. As new clinical research broaden our knowledge, change in programming and standards are required. All sources in this publication are believed to be reliable in their efforts to provide information that is complete and generally in accordance with the standards accepted at the time of publication. The suggestions recommended in the KT Diet 28-Day Meal Plan are not intended as a substitute for any exercise or dietary regimen prescribed by your doctor. As with any exercise and nutrition regiment, you should talk with your doctor and gain their approval before beginning any new program. Further, your doctor should perform an assessment of your overall health. It is important to note that any form of exercise or change in diet can have an inherent risk on a person's health. All readers are advised to take full responsibility for their actions and understand their limits. DRAEKK LLC, and the author hereby disclaim any liability or loss in connection with the use of this system, the dietary program, and advice herein.

Library of Congress Control Number (LCCN): 2018912676

ISBN: 978-0-692-04527-5

DRAEKK

It's Never Too Late To Become The Person You Were Meant To Be!
For more of our products, like the CONCEPT24® Planner, visit **draekk.com**

CONTENTS

THE BASICS

EVERYTHING YOU NEED TO KNOW

EVERYTHING YOU NEED TO KNOW

FOR YOUR KETO SUCCESS

INTRODUCTION

Get in the best shape of your life with the KT 28-Day Meal Plan! The new science in weight loss! The Ketogenic Diet (or keto) is a low-carb, high fat, and adequate protein diet that is scientifically proven to train your body to use stored fat as fuel. This natural process enables you to lose weight in a healthy, efficient and effective manner, providing you with clarity and energy...all without ever feeling hungry! This plan is developed by a Certified Personal Trainer and Fitness Nutrition Specialist. This meal plan was designed with your busy lifestyle in mind, you only have to cook 1-2 times per week! Most of the meals can be prepped and made during the weekend. No more wondering what to make for the week, it's already done for you. You can use this meal plan for 28 days, 3 months, or just a meal here and there to shake things up.

What You Get:
- 4 Weeks of Keto Meal Plans + Weekly Grocery Lists
- Specific Daily Meal Plans (What to Eat, How Much + When)
- All Macronutrients Calculated for You
- Nutritional Facts + Guidelines

WHAT IS KETO?

Although, keto is the new science in weight loss, the keto diet has been around since the 1920s as a proven treatment for epilepsy. It was first suggested by Dr. Russel Wilder in 1921 that a diet high in fat and low in carbs. could mimic the results of fasting. During a fasted state (or in the case of keto, a mimicked fasted state), the body goes through a metabolic adaptation (also known as ketosis), where the body uses stored fat as an energy source. Wilder proposed the ketogenic diet for his patients at the Mayo clinic and was able to report a significant reduction in seizers. Since then, the ketogenic diet is widely used as a treatment for epilepsy. Weight loss was noted as a side effect to the diet, thus prompting people to start using it as a viable weight loss system.

The keto diet is based on eating a specific percentage of macronutrients; Fat: 70-75%, Protein: 20-25%, Carbs.: 5%. In order to reach the metabolic state of ketosis, and for optimal weight loss potential, carb. intake is kept at 20 grams per day. All calculations are performed based off of carb. intake. If 20 grams of carbs. is 5% of your calories, then daily calorie allotment is 1600 calories. All the math has been done for you. This meal plan does allow for you to eat less or more based off your individual needs. The pyramid shows the general rule for keto macros.

KETO MACROS + PERCENTAGES

Your keto macro percentages are shown on the left and the subsequent grams (and calories) for each are shown on the right.

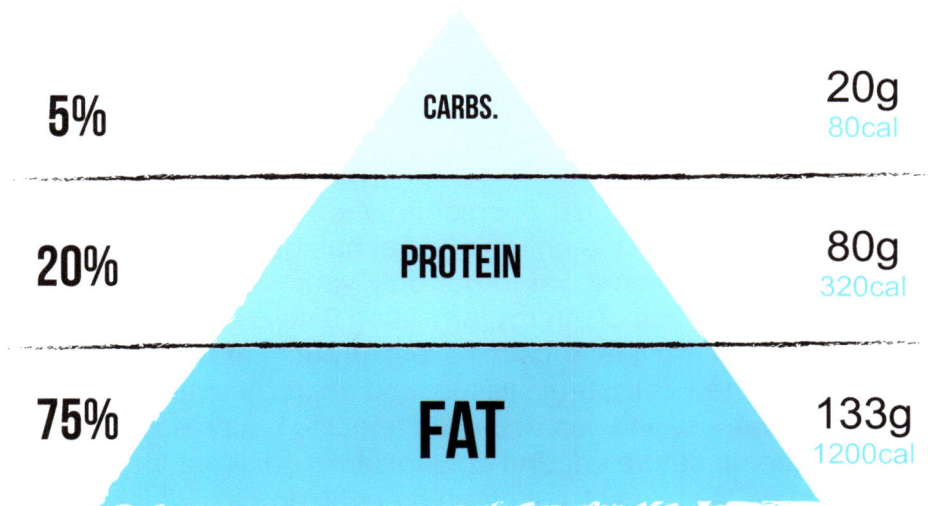

5%	CARBS.	20g 80cal
20%	PROTEIN	80g 320cal
75%	FAT	133g 1200cal

BASED ON 1600 CALORIE/DAY KETOGENIC DIET

WHAT IS THE KT DIET?

KT, or Keto Transformation, is exactly what it sounds like, it is the transformation your body and mind go through on a ketogenic diet. This plan takes your entire life into account, your busy schedule, your diet weaknesses, even your favorite foods. The KT Diet is all you need for weight loss success! One of the main reasons people fail on keto is because of all of the guesswork when it comes to meal prepping and calorie/macro counting. People spend hours on forums or Pinterest searching for a recipe that seems keto, but low and behold, it's not even low-carb. People have the intellectual capacity to understand how keto macros work, but make someone calculate every meal 2-3 times per day for months on end…it's a hard thing to stick to and frankly, it's way too much work. Well lucky you, you now have the proven KT 28-Day Meal Plan, the work is done for you. This book even addresses some of the rampant false information given by other keto 'authorities' in terms of adequate protein intake and the smokescreen of 'Net Carbs.'.

Join us and lose an average of 15 lbs. per month. It's time to take back control of your life.

LET'S TALK MACROS

Fats, carbohydrates, and proteins are the three macronutrients (or macros) essential to sustaining life. Fat provides 9 calories per gram, carbs. and protein each provide 4 calories per gram. Although, not an essential macro, alcohol is arguably a fourth macro, providing 7 calories per gram. The Keto Macros are: Fat: 70-75%, Protein: 20-25%, Carbs.: 5%.

FAT

One of the biggest hurdles people must overcome when embarking on keto is in dealing with the misconception that a fat-rich diet is unhealthy. Fat has been demonized for years, but recent research shows the keto diet is beneficial to not only your weight loss journey but your overall health as well. Fat is a great source of energy, providing 9 calories per gram, compared to protein and carbs., which each only provide 4 calories per gram. Fats are essential for many bodily functions, including making new cells, brain tissue, and neurotransmitters, it aids in the absorption of certain vitamins and minerals, and can act as an appetite suppressant. There are four types of fats: saturated, trans, monounsaturated, and polyunsaturated. Most foods contain a combination of the different types of fats. All fats are not created equal, on keto we embrace certain fats: olive oil, avocados, grass-fed meat, whole eggs, butter, omega 3s found in fatty fish, and medium-chain triglycerides (MCT) found in coconut oil, to name a few. Eating the recommended amount of fat will give you more energy and keep you satiated throughout the day. Getting the recommend amount of fat is vital to your keto success.

PROTEIN

Protein is important for proper growth and development. Each gram of protein provides 4 calories. The recommended daily intake of protein is .8 grams of protein for every 1 kilogram of body weight. **Remember that 1 kilogram equals 2.2 pounds.** Making the conversion from pounds to kilograms is vital. In the United States we have a problem, our scales measure our weight in pounds, not kilograms (this may be the reason why some of the 'leading keto authorities' forget to convert body weight in pounds to kilograms, thus advising keto goers everywhere to essentially double their recommended protein intake). Going over on protein intake will kick you out of ketosis. The next page has an example on how to calculate your recommended protein intake.

EXAMPLE: HOW MUCH PROTEIN DO YOU NEED?

How much protein(g) does a 180 lb. person need?

RECALL 1 KILOGRAM(KG) = 2.2 POUNDS(LBS.)

1. Convert bodyweight in pounds to kilograms.

$$180 \text{ lbs. } \times \frac{1 \text{ kg}}{2.2 \text{ lbs.}} = 81.8 \text{ kg}$$

2. Convert bodyweigh in kilograms to necessary protein intake in grams.

$$81.8 \text{ kg } \times \frac{.8 \text{ g}}{1 \text{ kg.}} = 65.5 \text{ g}$$

It is recommended a 180lb. person get 65.5 grams of protein per day.

KETO DIET PROTEIN MACROS ARE 20-25% OF DAILY CALORIC INTAKE

Okay, maybe you're not a mathematician, you just want to be told how to do the keto diet without the headache of all the math and macros. That is why we've done all the math for you and created the KT 28-Day Meal Plan, this plan is designed for optimum healthy weight loss in the most effective and efficient amount of time. NOTE: If you start to stall in your weight loss, one thing to try is to decrease your caloric intake. Decreasing your calories and sticking with the keto diet macros of **fat: 75%, protein: 20%, and carbs.: 5%,** your protein in grams will decrease as well.

RECOMMENDED PROTEIN INTAKE BY BODYWEIGHT

WEIGHT (LBS.)	WEIGHT (KGS.)	PROTEIN (G) INTAKE
300	136	109
250	114	90
200	91	73
180	82	65
150	68	55
130	59	47

CARBS.

Carbs. are found primarily in plant foods (with the exception of dairy products which contain lactose (milk sugar)). Each gram of carb. provides 4 calories. During digestion, carbs are converted into glucose (sugar), a good source of instant energy, however, most carbs. are not used right away, as they are not needed (unless for vigorous exercise). Those excess carbs. are stored as fat. There are several types of carbohydrates: sugar, starches, sugar alcohols, and fiber.

SUGAR: Sugar is quickly broken down into glucose. Excess sugar consumption has been attributed to certain cancers, obesity, Type 2 diabetes, non-alcoholic fatty liver disease, etc. Excess sugar should always be avoided. While doing keto, avoid any food with sugar listed in the nutrition label.

STARCHES: The majority of carbohydrates in a typical American diet are starches. Starches can be found in pasta, cereals, corn, flour, rice, potatoes, as well as most processed foods. While food manufactures must list fats, calories, total carbs., and fiber on nutrition labels, they are not required to list starches.

SUGAR ALCOHOLS: Sugar alcohols provide a sweet taste with fewer calories per gram than table sugar (sucrose), and are commonly used in place of sugar in food. Although foods made with sugar alcohols have less calories than foods made with sugar, they still provide calories and have been known to slow weight loss and most have an impact on blood glucose levels. Common sugar alcohols and their calories as stated by the US Food and Drug Administration (FDA): *Isomalt* (2 cal./g), *Lactitol* (2 cal./g), *Xylitol* (2.4 cal./g), *Maltitol* (2.1 cal./g), *Sorbitol* (2.6 cal./g), *Hydrogenated Starch Hydrolysates(HSH)* (3 cal./g), *Mannitol* (1.6 cal./g), *Erythritol* (0 cal./g).

FIBER: Dietary fiber, or fiber, is a type of carb. found in plant foods. Fiber has long been assumed to pass through the body without being digested, however, fiber isn't black or white; there are two types of fiber; soluble fiber and insoluble fiber.

- **Insoluble Fiber** (non-digestible fiber) does not dissolve in water and passes through the body mostly intact, aiding in bowel movements. It is not absorbed by the body, and therefore is not a source of calories.

- **Soluble Fiber** (partially digestible fiber) dissolves in water, and is broken down and fermented in the large intestine, it is partially absorbed and therefore provides some calories. The FDA states that a general factor of 2 calories per gram should be assigned for soluble fiber.

NET CARBS. OR TOTAL CARBS. - WHAT COUNTS?

It has long been a point of contention on whether people should count Total Carbs. or Net Carbs. The term Net Carbs. (aka 'impact carbs.' or 'effective carbs.') was coined by the food industry in the 70s as a way to market products as being low in carbs. The term is not legally recognized by the American Diabetes Association (ADA) or the US Food and Drug Administration (FDA). The food industry has long been using Net Carbs. as a smokescreen for hidden digestible carbs. The common myth in the low-carb community is that Fiber does not contribute to calorie count, which is only partially true, only Insoluble Fiber has zero calories, whereas Soluble Fiber provides some calories. Another misconception is that Sugar Alcohol does not contribute calories, when in actuality the only Sugar Alcohol that has zero calories is Erythritol. The blanket statement of calculating Net Carbs. by subtracting all Fiber and all Sugar Alcohol from Total Carbs. is inaccurate, dangerous, and quite misleading. Below is a more accurate guideline derived from the ADA and FDA to calculate carbs. that affect blood glucose levels (digestible carbs.). The KT Diet refers to digestible carbs. as Net Carbs. in the below equation.

- if food contains Sugar Alcohols, subtract half the Sugar Alcohol from Total Carbs.
- if the amount of Fiber in a serving of food is more than 5 grams, subtract half of the grams of Fiber from the Total Carbs.

$$\text{NET CARBS.} = \text{TOTAL CARBS.} - \tfrac{1}{2}(\text{FIBER})^* - \tfrac{1}{2}(\text{SUGAR ALCOHOLS})$$

*if the fiber quantity in food is more than 5 grams

Since ketosis is a fragile metabolic state, the carb. intake must be limited to 20 grams of digestible carbs. per day. It is up to you if you would like to calculate your carbs. based off of Total Carbs. or Net Carbs. (the correct calculation given in this book). Do not follow Net Carbs. from processed food labels, those labels have the high probability of hiding carbs. that do affect your blood glucose levels and can kick you out of ketosis. This meal plan calculates Net Carbs. based off of the guidelines derived from the ADA and FDA listed above.

SPECIAL CONCERNS

Whether you have Type 1 or Type 2 diabetes, are pregnant, have gestational diabetes, or are breastfeeding, it is always advisable to consult with your doctor prior to making any dietary changes.

- **PREGNANT OR BREASTFEEDING:** If you are pregnant or breastfeeding, it is not advisable to follow the keto diet. You will not receive enough of the recommended carbs. or nutrients. Pregnancy is not a time to experiment.
- **TYPE 2 DIABETIC:** Studies show that a keto diet can be effective in reducing key markers related to Type 2 diabetes, such as excess body weight and blood glucose (sugar) levels. The reduced amount of carbs. help eliminate large spikes in blood sugar, which can reduce the need for insulin. People with Type 2 diabetes that follow the keto diet need to carefully monitor their blood glucose levels, as they are at a higher risk of developing hypoglycemia (low blood sugar). For the most effective outcome, a doctor should be consulted to measure progress as well as adjust medication appropriately. The KT 28-Day Meal Plan has helped numerous Type 2 diabetics lose an average of 10 lbs. per month, while reducing the need for insulin.
- **TYPE 1 DIABETIC:** While management of Type 1 diabetes is outside the scope of this book, you can still consult with your doctor and a registered dietitian specializing in keto if you would like to implement this way of eating. Type 1 diabetics should be aware of diabetic ketoacidosis (DKA). This can be a life-threatening condition for people with Type 1 diabetes. This condition is not to be confused with nutritional ketosis (the safe fat burning state reached in the keto diet).

KETOSIS IS NOT KETOACIDOSIS

Despite the likeness in names, ketosis is not ketoacidosis. Ketosis refers to nutritional ketosis (the natural state your body enters during the keto diet). Ketosis is simply the natural process of producing small to moderate levels of ketones in the blood, which is not harmful. Whereas ketoacidosis refers to diabetic ketoacidosis, a serious complication of diabetes that occurs when the body produces an extremely high level of ketones that buildup in the blood, causing the blood to become acidic, which can alter the normal function of organs. Even if you do not have Type 1 diabetes and you are on the keto diet, you should still monitor ketone levels to make sure you have a healthy small to moderate level of ketones in the body.

EXERCISE

Exercise is the most transformative thing you can do for your body and mind. It is true that with the keto diet you can and will lose weight without exercise, however, the benefits you gain from adding in regular exercise has a great impact on your overall health. One of the main reasons for doing keto is to lose weight (fat specifically), but there is more to a healthy and happy life than just how you look. The point of dieting and exercising is feeling happy with the person that you are and the person that you are becoming. The best version of yourself is not solely about what you see in the mirror, but rather it is a compilation of your desired physical attributes and desired physical abilities.

Dieting is essential in losing weight, but exercise is essential in giving you a body that you can be active with. What are your dreams and aspirations, what things do you want to do in this life that require you to have a fully functioning body? Do you want to run a marathon, heck do you want to walk a marathon? Do you want to hike Machu Picchu, or maybe you just want to walk down the street without being winded. Whatever it is in life that you want to do, it requires a whole healthy body. You need to work on the whole system, your whole body, the diet will help with weight loss, but the exercising will give you strength and stamina. Start easy; crawl, walk, then run and take pride in knowing that you can take control and create an easy, fun, and effective exercise routine.

There are easy ways to get your exercise in; take the stairs instead of the elevator, take a walk at lunch or hit the gym, walk your dog a little further each day. There are many tips and tricks to encourage building a healthy exercise routine; leave your running shoes by the bed for a quick morning walk, or leave your gym clothes in the car so you have no excuse not to go to the gym after work. Make sure to avoid injury and increase flexibility by stretching before a workout. Make sure to track your goals and progress with the GOAL TRACKER at the back of this book.

Check out www.DRAEKK.com for workouts that are designed by a Certified Personal Trainer and are perfect for every workout level.

GOT GOALS. . . WE HAVE A PLANNER FOR THAT

If you have goals, then you need to plan for your success. The KT Meal Plan was designed in conjunction with The CONCEPT24® Planner, a planner with a proven weight loss system. With this day planner you can do it all, the daily pages give you a place to focus on your daily schedule as well as meal tracking, fitness, daily victories, even notes. Designed to help you break down your health goals into manageable monthly, weekly, and daily action tasks. Go to www.DRAEKK.com.

KETO SUCCESS
YOUR STEP-BY-STEP
GUIDE

KETO SUCCESS STEP-BY-STEP

STEP 1: REVIEW THIS BOOK AND TIPS

Are you ready to lose some weight? Well let's get started! This meal plan and guide was designed to be read in its entirety, each section has vital information for your weight loss success. This book will answer most questions you come across in the keto forums, from the basics on what the keto macros are, how much protein you need, to tips and tricks on how to get into and stay in ketosis, oh and of course how to lose weight! It's never wise to jump into something new without knowing the basics, so start at the beginning and work your way through.

STEP 2: REMOVE TEMPTATION

Giving in to temptation will make or break your diet. You may be able to exercise your willpower every once in a while, but at some point you will give in to temptation. Think of willpower like a muscle, it can fatigue with overuse. If you exercise your willpower too often, eventually you may find yourself giving in to temptation (aka the ice cream in the freezer). Set yourself up for success, get rid of anything non-keto friendly in the house, at the office, even car snacks. Go through your pantry, refrigerator, even your hidden stash of goodies (you know you have one somewhere), and get rid of all the non-keto approved foods. There is no need to test your willpower, if the food is in the house, you will find a reason to eat it. If it has carbs., give it away, bring it to the office breakroom, or throw it out!

If necessary, talk with loved ones, coworkers, and friends to give them a heads up as to your lifestyle change. You will have to work harder to make sure that your significant other or children do not derail your success. In some cases it is advisable to talk with your significant other about keeping certain tempting food out of the house in order to aid in your weight loss success. You may not gain the support that you desire, but this is about you and your health, not theirs. Be strong and keep at it, if you stick with this way of eating, you WILL get the body that you want and deserve.

STEP 3: GROCERY SHOP + MEAL PREP

A key factor in weight loss success is diet adherence, kinda obvious, right? You have to stick to a diet in order for it to work. The easiest way to adhere to any diet, is to meal prep. Meal prepping is not just for body builders or fitness fanatics, it is a vital strategy to implement in any diet. Cook once, eat for a week, this practice will free up your time and take the guesswork out of meal planning. Just dedicate a few weekend hours to making your food for the week, portion out your meals into individual Tupperware, then grab and go. The KT 28-Day Meal Plan is unique in that it is designed with your busy schedule in mind. Dieting is hard enough on its own, without having to cook a different meal each night. Just think of the nights when you get off work and are too tired to cook a full meal, you're more likely to grab something on the way home and potentially cheat on the diet. You have a better change of diet adherence if when you get home from work, the only thing you need to do is grab your already prepped food, heat and eat. The act of meal prepping will save you hours each night, essentially giving you back time.

Another unique advantage to the KT 28-Day Meal Plan is your food bill will go WAY DOWN. On this plan, people spend an average of $50 per week on food, and just think, you probably spent that in one day on dinner out, a fast food lunch, and a coffee and scone for breakfast, and don't forget the snack machine treats. This plan is unique in the world of keto meal plans, this plan does not require you to buy any fancy supplements, expensive keto powders or organics food, none of these are necessary for weight loss success (buying supplements and organic food is entirely up to the individual). Remember fatty meat is less expensive than lean meat; eggs, cheese, and veggies can be very reasonably priced and you do not need to go organic if you don't want to. So, if anyone tells you keto is expensive, tell them they're doing it wrong. With this plan you will not only lose weight, but you will also extensively lower your weekly food bill! Save that money and spend it on something fun, like your reward vacation for reaching your goal weight or that new wardrobe you will surely need!

STEP 4: GETTING INTO KETOSIS

Let's start losing weight! Okay, you've gone grocery shopping, prepped all the food, what's next? Well, you need to get into ketosis, lucky for you getting into ketosis is built into this meal plan, the only thing you need to do is follow the plan. If done properly, getting into ketosis should take anywhere from 2 - 7 days, although it can vary depending on how carb. dependent you were prior to the diet. In most cases weight loss should happen immediately as you are depriving your body or carbs. (the first few pounds are water weight, which is fine). The whole point of the keto diet is to get in the optimum state of ketosis, where you will not only lose weight, but feel more energetic as well. If you are new to keto, the first time you get into ketosis can feel a bit overwhelming, remember your body is using a new source of energy, so you may feel a bit off. That is why it is good to know the signs of when you are getting into ketosis, it will help motivate you. The initial stage of getting into ketosis is often referred to as the 'keto flu'.

KETO FLU

Keto flu, it's the talk of the town when it comes to starting keto, but it's not as bad as it sounds, as it can be avoided almost entirely with the right prep work and a well-balanced keto diet. So you may be wondering, what exactly is the keto flu and how can I avoid it? Glad you asked. During the first few days of starting the keto diet, you may experience headaches, fatigue, and brain fog. This combination of symptoms is deemed the keto flu. Keto flu symptoms usually only last 1 - 4 days. Luckily, you found the KT 28-Day Meal Plan, which is specifically designed to minimize the symptoms associated with the keto flu; the food and portion sizes have been designed to give you the proper nutrients to potentially avoid symptoms. However, even with a well-balanced keto meal plan, you may still experience some symptoms associated with the keto flu. It is a good idea to make sure you get enough potassium, magnesium, and sodium. Consult with your doctor to make sure you get the right amount of these as supplements. The keto flu should only last a few days, by which time your body becomes more adapted to using fat as energy and the keto flu symptoms will subside. Once in ketosis you will have an increase in energy, focus and a feeling of euphoria.

ARE YOU IN KETOSIS?

You need to remember that your body is going through changes on the keto diet, your body is learning to use a different, more efficient energy source (fat), so give your body time to adjust. Essentially your body is going through a carb. detox. Detoxing can have an effect on the body; during the first few weeks on keto some people have noted experiencing a few other subtle symptoms, such as keto breath, odd smelling sweat, fatigue, constipation (or diarrhea), excessive sweating, or odd smelling urine.

These symptoms are nothing to worry about, they are simply the natural process your body is going through to detox. If you have any of these symptoms, they do subside after a few weeks, when you become truly fat-adapted.

There are many ways to tell if you are in ketosis:

- **KETO BREATH:** During the initial stages of keto you may notice a distinct fruity or metallic taste in your mouth. When your body enters ketosis, your body creates the ketone bodies: acetone, acetoacetate, and beta hydroxybutyrate. Since ketones are expelled from the body through urination and exhalation, the distinct taste is caused by the exaltation of these ketones. Although, this may be unpleasant, it shows you are in ketosis and subsides after a few weeks.
- **KETO URINE TEST STRIPS:** An inexpensive way of checking if you are in ketosis, although they can be inaccurate, depending on your hydration levels (test in the morning after you are hydrated). Keto strips work best when you are first starting out on the keto diet, as your body will excrete a larger number of ketones in the beginning, before you have become fat-adapted. If you are in ketosis, the strip will change colors from its original beige, the darker the color, the deeper you are into ketosis. A good range to shoot for is low to midrange on the guide. Be aware that a deep deep purple color can mean you are dehydrated.
- **KETO BREATH METER:** Another alternative to check if you are in ketosis is by using a keto breath meter. With this method you are measuring the level of ketones in your breath. Results are generally more accurate than with Keto Urine Test Strips, but still not as accurate as testing for ketosis with a Blood Meter.
- **KETO BLOOD METER:** The most accurate (and most expensive) way to measure if you are in ketosis. It measures the ketone levels in blood rather than in urine or breath. If you are in ketosis, the Keto Blood Meter should measure between 0.5 – 3 mmol/L. Values of 3mmol/L are not necessary to achieve optimal ketosis.

STEP 5: MAINTAINING KETOSIS

Simply follow the base meal plan provided in this book and you will stay in ketosis. If you are doing this diet to lose weight, it is advisable to record your weight, make sure to check the scale every day at the same time (the best time is in the morning after you have gone to the restroom and prior to eating). It is possible to be in ketosis and not lose weight, this usually only happens months into keto. If you are in ketosis and you are not losing weight it could signify that it is time to reduce your caloric intake (the less you weigh the less calories you need) or that you may be getting too many carbs. (make sure to follow the 'Net Carb.' calculations in this book, so as to avoid hidden carbs). Make sure to keep carbs. at or below 20 grams per day. Checking the scale every day will give you insight into what is and what is not working. With keto, the scale is no longer the enemy, but your new best friend, congratulating you on your hard work and giving you good news each morning!

KETO SUCCESS TIPS

TIP
1 | REMOVE
TEMPTATIONS

Go through your pantry, refrigerator, even your hidden stash of goodies (you know you have one hidden somewhere), and get rid of all the non-keto approved foods. There is no need to test your willpower, if the food is in the house, you will find a reason to eat it. If it has carbs., give it away, bring it to the office breakroom, or throw it out!

TIP
2 | MEAL
PREP

This meal plan is designed with your busy schedule in mind, you do not have time to make a different meal every night. Cook once, eat for a week, this practice will free up your time and take the guesswork out of meal planning. Dedicate a few weekend hours to making your food for the week, then just grab and go.

TIP
3 | DO NOT
CHEAT!!!

You will not succeed if you give in to temptations, do not have any sweets, chips, or other non-keto approved snacks in the house. If you cheat, you will most likely be kicked out of ketosis, and in most cases it will take about a week to get back into ketosis, which means you miss out on a whole week of weight loss. Do not cheat, it is not worth it!

TIP
4 | HAVE KETO
SNACKS ON HAND

Let's be honest, even if you plan everything out, things can still go wrong during the day, and you may be tempted to cheat. You may get stuck in a meeting, kids practice runs long, you name it. That is why having keto approved snacks on hand will save you. Check out the Keto Approved Snacks (pg. 75) and pick a few to keep on hand.

TIP
5 | DON'T EAT
TOO MUCH PROTEIN

The protein amount specified on the keto diet is kept moderate at 20% of your calories, enough to preserve lean body mass, while still allowing you to enter ketosis. However, eating too much protein can prevent ketosis, as the amino acids in protein can be converted to glucose (sugar), a process called gluconeogenesis. Your body may utilize that new sugar as an energy source (fuel) versus using your own stored body fat (the purpose of keto). Too much protein could keep you from losing the optimum amount of weight in the most efficient amount of time.

TIP 6 | GET ENOUGH FATS

Keto is a high fat diet, 75% of your calories come from fat. Fats are essential for most bodily functions, including making new cells, brain tissue, and neurotransmitters. Eating the recommended amount of fat will give you more energy and keep you satiated throughout the day. Getting the recommend amount of fat will help you be successful.

TIP 7 | DRINK ENOUGH WATER

When you significantly reduce your carb. intake, your glycogen (sugar) stores are depleted. Each gram of glycogen stores 3 grams of water, when those stores are depleted, the kidneys excrete more water. As a result, the initial weight lost during keto is water weight. The downside is that with additional water excreted, you will lose additional electrolytes. Dehydration is a common side effect on keto, therefore make sure you drink a gallon of water per day.

TIP 8 | GET YOUR ELECTROLYTES

Even with a well-formulated keto diet and enough water, you may still experience headaches, muscle cramps, and other keto flu like symptoms. Help avoid these and other symptoms, by ensuring you balance the electrolytes in your system. Electrolytes are critical on the keto diet, make sure you get enough potassium, sodium and magnesium.

TIP 9 | START WITH THE BASICS, THEN EXPERIMENT

Do not sabotage your success by trying too many things at once. Start with this easy to do and effective meal plan, then when your body has adjusted and you are comfortable with this way of eating, you can branch out and potentially add other dieting methods to your weight loss repertoire. Make sure to only add one thing at a time, that way you can determine what is helping or hindering your success. You do not need to try intermittent fasting or expensive supplements when you are first starting out. Keep it simple and succeed.

TIP 10 | MEASURE YOUR GOALS

If you have goals, then you need to plan for your success. The KT Diet Meal Plan was designed in conjunction with The CONCEPT24® Planner, a planner with a proven weight loss system. With this day planner you can do it all, the daily pages give you a place to focus on your daily schedule as well as meal tracking, fitness, daily victories, even notes. Designed to help you break down your health goals into manageable monthly, weekly, and daily action tasks. You can even track your body composition to see your progress. Go to www.DRAEKK.com or see more information at the back of this book on how to get a discount on your CONCEPT24® Planner.

COMMON FOOD CARB. COUNT

Avoid hidden carbs. Each item is listed with its accompanying serving size, Total Carbs., Fiber, and Net Carbs. (in grams). The American Diabetes Association and FDA give guidelines on how to calculate the carb. count based off of the digestible carbs: *if the quantity of Fiber in a food is more than 5 grams (per serving), subtract half of the grams of Fiber from the Total Carbs.*

FOOD	SERVINGS	TOTAL CARBS. (g)	FIBER (g)	NET CARBS. (g)
WHITE BREAD	1 Slice	21	1.4	21
BUN (HAMBURGER)	1	25	< 1	25
ENGLISH MUFFIN	1	24	< 1	24
PANCAKE	1 (10" diameter)	60	3	60
TORTILLA (CORN)	1 (7" diameter)	10.7	1.3	10.7
WAFFLE (FROZEN)	1 (4" diameter)	16	< 1	16
BEANS (REFRIED) CANNED	½ cup	16.1	4.4	16.1
OATMEAL (STEEL CUT, DRY)	¼ cup	27	4	27
WHITE ALL-PURPOSE FLOUR, ENRICHED	1 cup	95	4	95
PASTA , SPAGHETTI (COOKED)	1 cup	46.6	2.7	46.6
RICE (COOKED)	1 cup	44.5	< 1	44.5
PIZZA (PEPPERONI)	1 slice	35	2.9	35
CORN	½ cup	11.8	1.6	11.8
PEAS	½ cup	11.4	3.6	11.4
POTATOES (MASHED)	1 cup	44.1	4.4	44.1
BROCCOLI (CHOPPED)	1 cup	11.2	5.1	8.7
CUCUMBER (WITH PEEL)	1 (medium)	7.8	2.5	7.8
ZUCCHINI (COOKED)	1 (medium)	4.5	1.7	4.5
CARROT (RAW)	1 (medium)	5.8	1.7	5.8
WHITE ONION (CHOPPED / COOKED)	1 cup	21.3	2.9	21.3
SPINACH (RAW / CHOPPED)	1 cup	1.1	< 1	1.1
ROMAINE LETTUCE	3 leaves	3	2	3
CAULIFLOWER (CHOPPED / COOKED)	1 cup	5.1	2.9	5.1
ASPARAGUS SPEARS	5 (medium)	3	1.5	3

FOOD	SERVINGS	TOTAL CARBS. (g)	FIBER (g)	NET CARBS. (g)
2 % MILK (COW)	1 cup	12	0	12
EGG	1	0.4	0	0.4
YOGURT (PLAIN / WHOLE MILK)	1 cup	11.4	0	11.4
CREAM CHEESE	1 Tbsp.	0.8	0	0.8
SOUR CREAM	1 Tbsp.	0.7	0	0.7
HEAVY CREAM	1 Tbsp.	0.4	0	0.4
AVOCADO	1 (medium)	11.8	9.2	7.2
APPLE	1 (medium)	25.1	4.4	25.1
BANANA	1 (medium)	27	3.1	27
STRAWBERRY	1 (medium)	1	0.2	1
GRAPES (SEEDLESS)	1	1	0	1
ORANGE	1 (medium)	15.4	3.1	15.4
BLUEBERRIES	1	0.2	0	0.2
APPLE JUICE	1 cup	29	0.2	29
ORANGE JUICE	1 cup	25.8	0.5	25.8
COKE / PEPSI	1 can (12oz.)	39 / 41	0 / 0	39 / 41
MILKSHAKE (VANILLA)	16 oz.	99.9	0	99.9
BEER	1 bottle (12oz.)	12.7	0	12.7
WINE (RED)	1 glass (5oz.)	4	0	4
DONUT (CHOCOLATE FROSTED)	1	31	1	31
CUPCAKE	1	30.3	1.4	30.3
FRENCH FRIES	1 (small)	30.3	3.1	30.3
TORTILLA CHIPS	1	1.4	0.1	1.4
DARK CHOCOLATE	1 oz.	13	3.1	13
ALMONDS	1	0.3	0.2	0.3
PEANUT BUTTER	1 Tbsp.	4.5	1	4.5
BBQ SAUCE	1 Tbsp.	7.1	0.2	7.1
KETCHUP	1 Tbsp.	4.1	0	4.1
RANCH	1 Tbsp.	0.5	0	0.5

WEEKLY MEAL PLANS

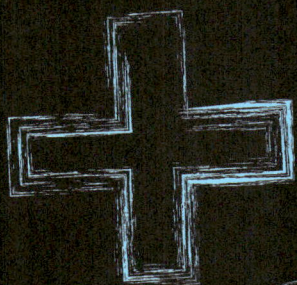

+ SHOPPING LISTS

WEEK 1 MEAL PLAN
AND SNACK OPTIONS

NUTRITION (DAILY): WITH EGG SALAD LUNCH
Calories: 1570; **Fat:** 130g (1170cal); **Protein:** 80g (320cal); **Net Carbs:** 20g (80cal)
NUTRITION (DAILY): WITH CHICKEN SALAD LUNCH
Calories: 1297; **Fat:** 101g (909cal); **Protein:** 79g (316cal); **Net Carbs.:** 18g (72cal)

NET CARBS = TOTAL CARBS - ½(FIBER*) - ½(SUGAR ALCOHOLS)
* if there is more than 5 grams of fiber in one serving, subtract half of it (not all of it)

The Net Carbs were calculated based off of the individual recipes. To alter any recipe or portion size check the individual recipes.

MORNING DRINK:
Detox Drink (warm or cold) (pg. 77)

BREAKFAST:
1 Oh So Cheesy Sausage Egg Muffin (pg. 40)
2 Slices Bacon
1 CUP Keto Coffee Bulletproof Style (pg. 81) (Optional: Can replace with Keto Coffee pg. 80)

SNACK (AM): ONLY IF NECESSARY
1 String Cheese (pg. 75)

LUNCH:
½ **CUP** Keto Egg Salad (pg. 65) **OR** ½ **CUP** Keto Chicken Salad (pg. 64)
1 Slice Bacon
1 Piece Romaine Lettuce

SNACK (PM): ONLY IF NECESSARY.
3 Pepperoni Slices + 3 Cubes of Cheese (1/2 inch.) (pg. 75)

DINNER:
1½ CUPS Keto Kickstart Soup (pg. 49)

DESSERT: ONLY IF NECESSARY.
Choose one from Keto Approved Snack Section (pg. 75) or Drinks + Desserts Section (pg. 76-83)

If you make any substitutions or add keto approved snacks make sure to track the additional calories.

WEEK 1 SHOPPING LIST

This shopping list is designed so you only need to buy what you need each week. Make sure to look at your snack options and add your choices to your weekly shopping list.

PRODUCE

1 Head	Romaine Lettuce
1	White Onion
1 Jar	Garlic (minced)
1 Bunch	Celery
1 Packet	Sun Dried Tomatoes
1 Head	Cauliflower
1 Bunch	Swiss / Rainbow Chard (may use Kale or Spinach)
1	Yellow Squash
1 Package	Fresh Green Beans (or canned)

REFRIGERATED

1 Dozen Large	Eggs
Small Container	Liquid Egg Whites
1 Pint	Heavy Cream
1 Bag (7-8oz)	Cheddar Cheese (Shredded)
1 Jar	Real Mayonnaise
2-4 Sticks	Butter
1 Pack	String Cheese
1 Block	Cheese Of Choice (or 1/2" Cubed)

MEAT

6 oz.	Breakfast Sausage (Ground)
3 - 12oz. Packages	Bacon
2	Chicken Breasts
2 - 5 oz (2 Cans)	Canned Chicken Breast (in Water)
1 Package	Pepperoni Slices

HERBS/SPICES

	Salt / Pepper
	Cayenne Pepper
	Mustard

OTHER

3 - 32 oz Cartons	Chicken Broth/ Stock
	Olive Oil
	MCT Oil
	Real Lemon Juice
	Coffee (No Sugar)
	Liquid Stevia Drops (Optional)

WEEK 2 MEAL PLAN
AND SNACK OPTIONS

NUTRITION (DAILY):

Calories: 1370; **Fat:** 114g (1026cal); **Protein:** 67g (269cal); **Net Carbs:** 18.8g (75cal)

NET CARBS = TOTAL CARBS - ½(FIBER*) - ½(SUGAR ALCOHOLS)
* if there is more than 5 grams of fiber in one serving, subtract half of it (not all of it)

The Net Carbs were calculated based off of the individual recipes. To alter any recipe or portion check the individual recipes.

MORNING DRINK:
Detox Drink (warm or cold) (pg. 77)

BREAKFAST:
Eggs Popeye (pg. 42)
1 CUP Keto Coffee Bulletproof Style (pg. 81) (Optional: *Can replace with Keto Coffee pg. 80*)

SNACK (AM): ONLY IF NECESSARY
Choose one from Keto Approved Snack Section (pg. 75)

LUNCH:
1¼ CUP Broccoli Cheddar Cauliflower Soup *(pg. 51)*

SNACK (PM): ONLY IF NECESSARY.
Choose one from Keto Approved Snack Section (pg. 75)

DINNER:
Next Level Stuffed Chicken ½ Stuffed Chicken Breast (pg. 55-56)
Green Salad w/ Ranch (pg. 73)

DESSERT: ONLY IF NECESSARY.
Choose one from Keto Approved Snack Section (pg. 75) or Drinks + Desserts Section (pg. 76-83)

If you make any substitutions or add keto approved snacks make sure to track the additional calories.

WEEK 2 SHOPPING LIST

This shopping list is designed so you only need to buy what you need each week. Make sure to look at your snack options and add your choices to your weekly shopping list.

PRODUCE

1 Bag	Spinach
1 Bunch	Celery
1 Jar	Garlic (minced)
1 Head	Cauliflower
1 Head	Broccoli (or 1 Bag Fresh)
1 Bag	Mixed Salad Greens

REFRIGERATED

1 Dozen Large	Eggs
2-4 Sticks	Butter
1 Pint	Heavy Cream
1 Bag (7-8oz)	Cheddar Cheese (Shredded)
1 Bag (7-8oz)	Mozzarella Cheese (Shredded)
1 Bag (7-8oz)	Parmesan Cheese (Shredded/Grated)
2 - 8 oz Packages	Cream Cheese
1 Bottle	Ranch Dressing (Less than 2g carb/serv)

MEAT

1 - 12oz. Package	Bacon
4	Large Chicken Breasts

HERBS/SPICES

Salt / Pepper

Cayenne Pepper

Cinnamon

Garlic Powder

Onion Powder

OTHER

2 - 32 oz Cartons	Chicken Broth/Stock
	Olive Oil
	Real Lemon Juice
	Liquid Stevia Drops (Optional)
	MCT Oil
	Coffee (No Sugar)
	Bag of Pork Rinds

WEEK 3 MEAL PLAN
AND SNACK OPTIONS

NUTRITION (DAILY):

Calories: 1348; **Fat:** 108g (972cal); **Protein:** 74g (296cal); **Net Carbs:** 20g (80cal)

NET CARBS = TOTAL CARBS - ½(FIBER*) - ½(SUGAR ALCOHOLS)
* if there is more than 5 grams of fiber in one serving, subtract half of it (not all of it)

The Net Carbs were calculated based off of the individual recipes. To alter any recipe or portion check the individual recipes.

MORNING DRINK:
Detox Drink (warm or cold) (pg. 77)

BREAKFAST:
1 Quiche Lorraine (pg. 41)
1 Slice Bacon
1 CUP Keto Coffee (pg. 80) (Optional)

SNACK (AM): ONLY IF NECESSARY
Choose one from Keto Approved Snack Section (pg. 75)

LUNCH:
1 CUP Zuppa Toscana (pg. 47)

SNACK(PM): ONLY IF NECESSARY.
Choose one from Keto Approved Snack Section (pg. 75)

DINNER:
Chicken Alfredo A'La Keto (pg. 59)
½ Chicken Breast, ½ **CUP** Spaghetti Squash, ¼ **CUP** Alfredo Sauce
Green Salad w/ Olive Oil and Cucumber (pg. 73)

DESSERT: ONLY IF NECESSARY.
Choose one from Keto Approved Snack Section (pg. 75) or Drinks + Desserts Section (pg. 76-83)

If you make any substitutions or add keto approved snacks make sure to track the additional calories.

WEEK 3 SHOPPING LIST

This shopping list is designed so you only need to buy what you need each week. Make sure to look at your snack options and add your choices to your weekly shopping list.

PRODUCE

1	Large Spaghetti Squash
1	White Onion
1 Jar	Garlic (minced)
1 Bag	Spinach
1 Bag	Mixed Salad Greens
1 Head	Cauliflower
1 Bunch	Swiss / Rainbow Chard (may use Kale or Spinach)
1	Cucumber

REFRIGERATED

1 Dozen Large	Eggs
Small Container	Liquid Egg Whites
2 Pints	Heavy Cream
1 Bag (7-8oz)	Swiss Cheese (Shredded)
1 Bag (7-8oz)	Parmesan Cheese (Shredded)
1 Stick	Butter

MEAT

1 lb.	Italian Sausage Spicy/Mild
2 - 12oz. Packages	Bacon
4	Large Chicken Breasts

HERBS/SPICES

- Salt / Pepper
- Cayenne Pepper
- Red Pepper Flakes
- Italian Seasonings
- Onion Powder

OTHER

2 - 32 oz Cartons	Chicken Broth/Stock
	Olive Oil
	MCT Oil
	Real Lemon Juice
	Coffee (No Sugar)
	Liquid Stevia Drops (Optional)

WEEK 4 MEAL PLAN
AND SNACK OPTIONS

NUTRITION (DAILY):

Calories: 1412; **Fat:** 108g (972cal); **Protein:** 90g (360cal); **Net Carbs:** 20g (80cal)

NET CARBS = TOTAL CARBS - ½(FIBER*) - ½(SUGAR ALCOHOLS)
* if there is more than 5 grams of fiber in one serving, subtract half of it (not all of it)

The Net Carbs were calculated based off of the individual recipes. To alter any recipe or portion check the individual recipes.

MORNING DRINK:
Detox Drink (warm or cold) (pg. 77)

BREAKFAST:
Mexi-Cali Scrambled Eggs (pg. 43)
1 Slice Bacon
1 CUP Keto Coffee (pg. 80) (Optional)

SNACK (AM): ONLY IF NECESSARY
Choose one from Keto Approved Snack Section (pg. 75)

LUNCH:
1¼ CUPS Keto Albondigas Soup (pg. 53)

SNACK(PM): ONLY IF NECESSARY.
Choose one from Keto Approved Snack Section (pg. 75)

DINNER:
½ **CUP CUT** Perfect Pork Roast + ¼ **CUP** Keto Gravy (pg. 63)
½ **CUP** Cheesy Mashed Cauliflower (pg. 72)
½ **CUP CUT** Parmesan Roasted Green Beans (pg. 70) (*May replace with Asparagus pg. 71*)
(Will have to make a second batch mid-way through the week).

DESSERT: ONLY IF NECESSARY.
Choose one from Keto Approved Snack Section (pg. 75) or Drink + Desserts Section (pg. 76-83)

If you make any substitutions or add keto approved snacks make sure to track the additional calories.

WEEK 4 SHOPPING LIST

This shopping list is designed so you only need to buy what you need each week. Make sure to look at your snack options and add your choices to your weekly shopping list.

PRODUCE

1	Zucchini
1	White Onion
1 Jar	Garlic (minced)
1 Bunch	Cilantro
1 Bunch	Celery
1	Tomato
24 oz.	Green Beans (may use Asparagus)
1 Head	Cauliflower

REFRIGERATED

1 Dozen Large	Eggs
8 oz	Sour Cream
1 Pint	Heavy Cream
1 Jar	Salsa (Less than 2g carb/serv)
1 Bag (7-8oz)	Parmesan Cheese (Shredded)
1 Bag (7-8oz)	Pepper Jack Cheese Or Preferred (Shredded)
1 Stick	Butter

MEAT

3-4lb.	Pork Shoulder Roast (Boneless)
1 lb.	Ground Beef (80/20)
1 - 12oz. Packages	Bacon

HERBS/SPICES

- Salt / Pepper
- Cayenne Pepper
- Ground Cumin
- Italian Seasonings
- Oregano
- Garlic Powder
- Rosemary

OTHER

2 - 32 oz Cartons	Chicken Broth/Stock
	Olive Oil
	MCT Oil
	Real Lemon Juice
	Coffee (No Sugar)
	Liquid Stevia Drops (Optional)

RECIPES

28 day's worth of keto-licious food. This plan is unique in that it has base nutritional information; you have a base meal plan and you can add snacks and desserts as you deem necessary. The Week 1 Meal Plan has snacks built in to help with the transition into keto. Week 2 - 4 do not have snacks or desserts included in the base meal plans, although you have the option to add any of the keto approved snacks and desserts from this cookbook. The KT 28-Day Meal Plan is all about options, simply look at the base meal plan for the week and add in extras as you feel fit. Make sure to record your additional calories and stay within your macros.

It is important to note that snacks and desserts are not necessary and only add if absolutely need to. Remember this is your health and your weight loss journey, so exercise caution with snacks and desserts.

BE DISCIPLINED...EVERYTHING IN MODERATION

BREAKFAST

OH SO CHEESY SAUSAGE EGG MUFFINS

Nothing screams brunch like quiche! From our healthy kitchen to yours, we bring you the guiltless, crust-less, oh so cheesy sauage and egg muffin. Kill the carbs and embrace flavor. Without the crust this is a perfect quick grab-n-go breakfast or snack with minimal carbs.

SERVINGS: 12 | SERVING SIZE: 1 QUICHE

INGREDIENTS

- **6 oz. breakfast sausage (cooked and crumbled)**
- **3 eggs**
- **5 egg whites**
- **1 cup heavy cream**
- **1 cup cheddar cheese (shredded)**
- **½ tsp. pepper**
- **½ tsp. salt**

STEPS

1. Preheat oven to 375 degrees F.

2. In a large mixing bowl mix eggs, egg whites, heavy cream, pepper, and salt.

3. Grease muffin tin. Divide the cheese and sausage among the 12 muffin cups.

4. Ladle enough egg mixture into each muffin cup to fill about 2/3 full.

5. Bake for 15-30 minutes (depending on size of muffin tin).

6. Enjoy this quick-grab, low-carb breakfast every morning! Refrigerate for up to 7 days. Heat for 25-35 sec. in microwave.

NUTRITION (PER SERV.): 1 QUICHE
Calories: 198; **Fat:** 17.3g; **Protein:** 9g; **Total Carbs:** 1.6g
Fiber: 0g, Net Carbs: 1.6g

NET CARBS = TOTAL CARBS - ½(FIBER*) - ½(SUGAR ALCOHOLS)
* if there is more than 5 grams of fiber in one serving, subtract half of it (not all of it)

MINI QUICHE LORRAINE MUFFINS

Although, quiche is now considered a classic French dish, it actually originated in Germany. The Germans originally called it 'kuchen,' meaning cake, and the French later renamed it 'Lorraine,' named after the Lorraine region of France. This keto friendly and universally appealing brunch combination is ideal for any occasion.

SERVINGS: 12 | SERVING SIZE: 1 QUICHE

INGREDIENTS

- **6 oz. bacon (cooked and crumbled)**
- **½ cup chopped white onion**
- **1 Tbsp. olive oil**
- **3 eggs**
- **5 egg whites**
- **1 cup heavy cream**
- **1 cup shredded Swiss cheese**
- **½ cup chopped spinach (destemmed)**
- **½ tsp. pepper**
- **½ tsp. salt**

STEPS

1. Preheat oven to 375 degrees F.

2. In a large mixing bowl mix eggs, egg whites, heavy cream, pepper, and salt.

3. Grease muffin tin. Divide the cheese, onions, spinach, and bacon among the 12 muffin cups.

4. Ladle enough egg mixture into each muffin cup to fill about 2/3 full.

5. Bake for 15-30 minutes (depending on size of muffin tin).

6. Enjoy this quick-grab, low-carb breakfast every morning! Refrigerate for up to 7 days. Heat for 25-35 sec. in microwave.

NUTRITION (PER SERV.): 1 QUICHE
Calories: 162; **Fat:** 13.7g; **Protein:** 7.6g; **Total Carbs:** 2g
Fiber: 0.3g, Net Carbs: 2g

NET CARBS = TOTAL CARBS - ½(FIBER*) - ½(SUGAR ALCOHOLS)

* if there is more than 5 grams of fiber in one serving, subtract half of it (not all of it)

EGGS POPEYE

Everyone knows the infamous Popeye, with his odd accent, strength of an ox, and a legendary love of spinach. The cartoon was created in the 1920s with a side agenda to highlight the health benefits of spinach. The ever so popular Popeye was subsequently credited with a 33 percent increase in U.S. spinach consumption. This dish is a shout-out to Popeye; sautéed spinach, crispy bacon, eggs, and cream cheese partner perfectly to create a healthy and bold keto breakfast.

SERVINGS: 1

INGREDIENTS

- 1 slice bacon (cooked + crumbled)
- 1 egg
- ½ Tbsp. butter
- ½ Tbsp. cream cheese
- ¼ cup spinach (chopped)
- pinch salt

STEPS

1. Melt butter in skillet on medium heat.

2. Add crumbled bacon.

3. Add spinach and saute.

4. Whisk eggs, add salt, then add to skillet.

5. Cut cream cheese into small amounts and stir into egg mixture.

6. Stir everything together, then enjoy!

NUTRITION (PER SERV.): 1 SERVING
Calories: 199; **Fat:** 16g; **Protein:** 11g; **Total Carbs:** 2.7g
Fiber: 1.1g, Net Carbs: 2.7g

NET CARBS = TOTAL CARBS - ½(FIBER*) - ½(SUGAR ALCOHOLS)
* if there is more than 5 grams of fiber in one serving, subtract half of it (not all of it)

MEXI-CALI SCRAMBLED EGGS

This quick and easy, colorful scramble will take you south of the border with the flavors of Mexico in every bite. The trick to the perfect scramble is to scramble the eggs until it starts to set, then remove skillet from heat, and allow the dish to finish cooking from residual heat.

SERVINGS: 1

INGREDIENTS

- **1 slice bacon (cooked + crumbled)**
- **1 egg**
- **½ Tbsp. butter**
- **1 Tbsp. sour cream**
- **1 Tbsp. salsa**
- **pinch salt**

STEPS

1. Melt butter in skillet on medium heat.
2. Add crumbled bacon.
3. Whisk eggs, add salt, then add to skillet.
4. Stir in sour cream and salsa into egg mixture.

NUTRITION (PER SERV.): 1 SERVING
Calories: 147; **Fat:** 11g; **Protein:** 9.6g; **Total Carbs:** 2.4g
Fiber: 0.3g, Net Carbs: 2.4g

NET CARBS = TOTAL CARBS - ½(FIBER*) - ½(SUGAR ALCOHOLS)
* if there is more than 5 grams of fiber in one serving, subtract half of it (not all of it)

MAINS

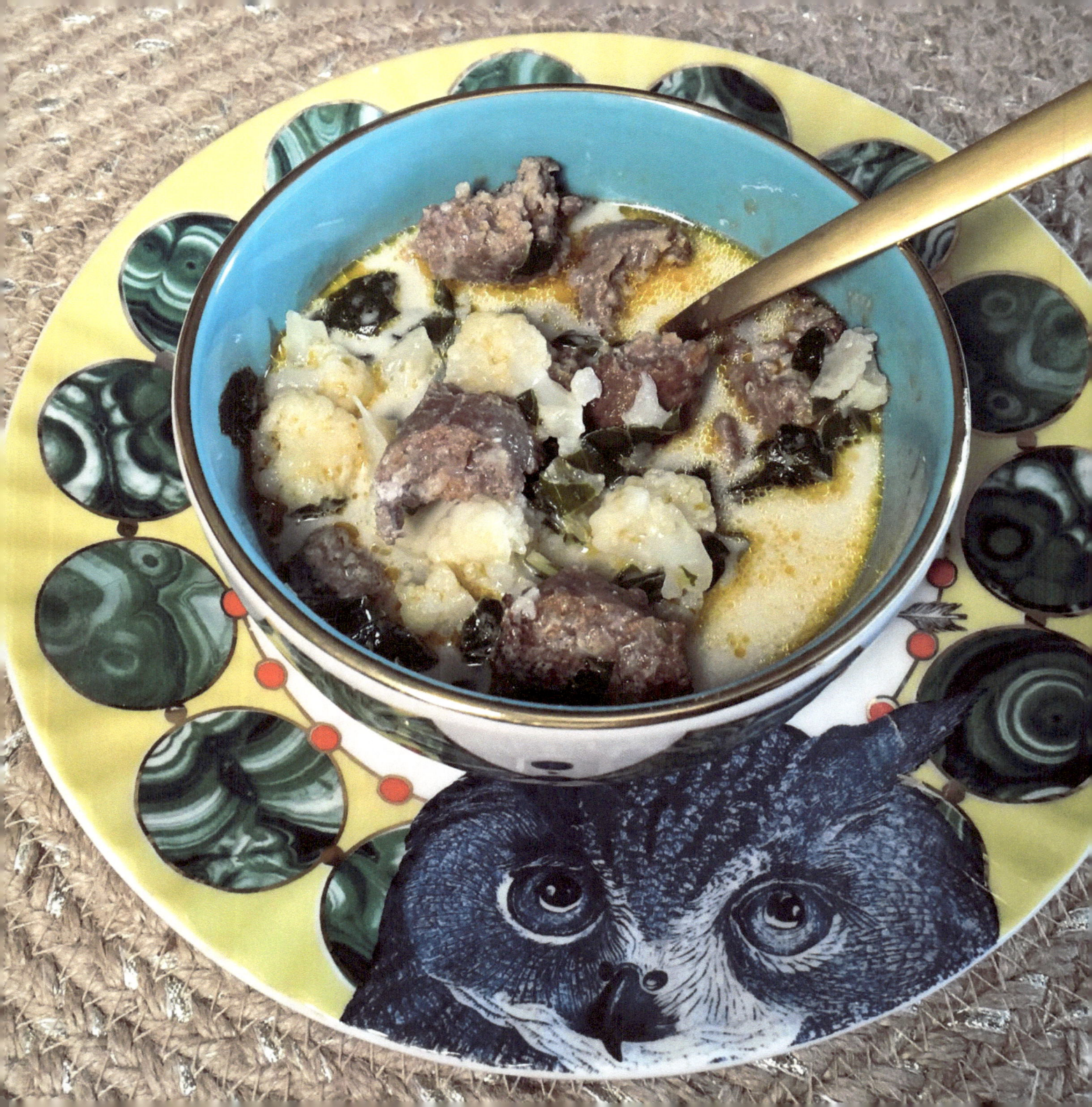

ZUPPA TOSCANA
OH SO SLIGHTLY SPICY
SAUSAGE CAULIFLOWER
SOUP

You're sure to melt the snow with this slightly spicy soup. This dish features the distinct flavors of Italy, a rich cream sauce and Italian sausage, blended with cauliflower and chard to create a flavor explosion. You're sure to be transported to the canals of Venice on a cold winter day, enjoying some of the local cuisine.

SERVINGS: 7 | SERVING SIZE: 1 CUP

INGREDIENTS

- **6 cups chicken stock or broth**
- **1 cup heavy cream**
- **1 head cauliflower**
- **4 cups chopped chard**
- **1 lb. spicy/mild Italian Sausage**
- **½ tsp. salt**
- **½ tsp. red pepper flakes** (optional)

STEPS

1. Grill or sauté the sausage per packaging. Crumble or cut the sausage into pieces.

2. While cooking sausage, combine the stock and cream in a saucepan over medium heat.

3. Crumble the cauliflower and cut the chard into small pieces. Add to the soup.

4. Add the sausage, salt and crushed red pepper flakes to the soup and simmer for 1 hour. Stir occasionally.

5. Serve and enjoy this slightly spicy winter warm up!

NOTE: May use kale or spinach if chard is not available.

NUTRITION (PER SERV.): 1 CUP
Calories: 310; **Fat:** 24g; **Protein:** 16.4g; **Total Carbs:** 10g
Fiber: 6g, Net Carbs: 7g

NET CARBS = TOTAL CARBS - ½(FIBER*) - ½(SUGAR ALCOHOLS)
* if there is more than 5 grams of fiber in one serving, subtract half of it (not all of it)

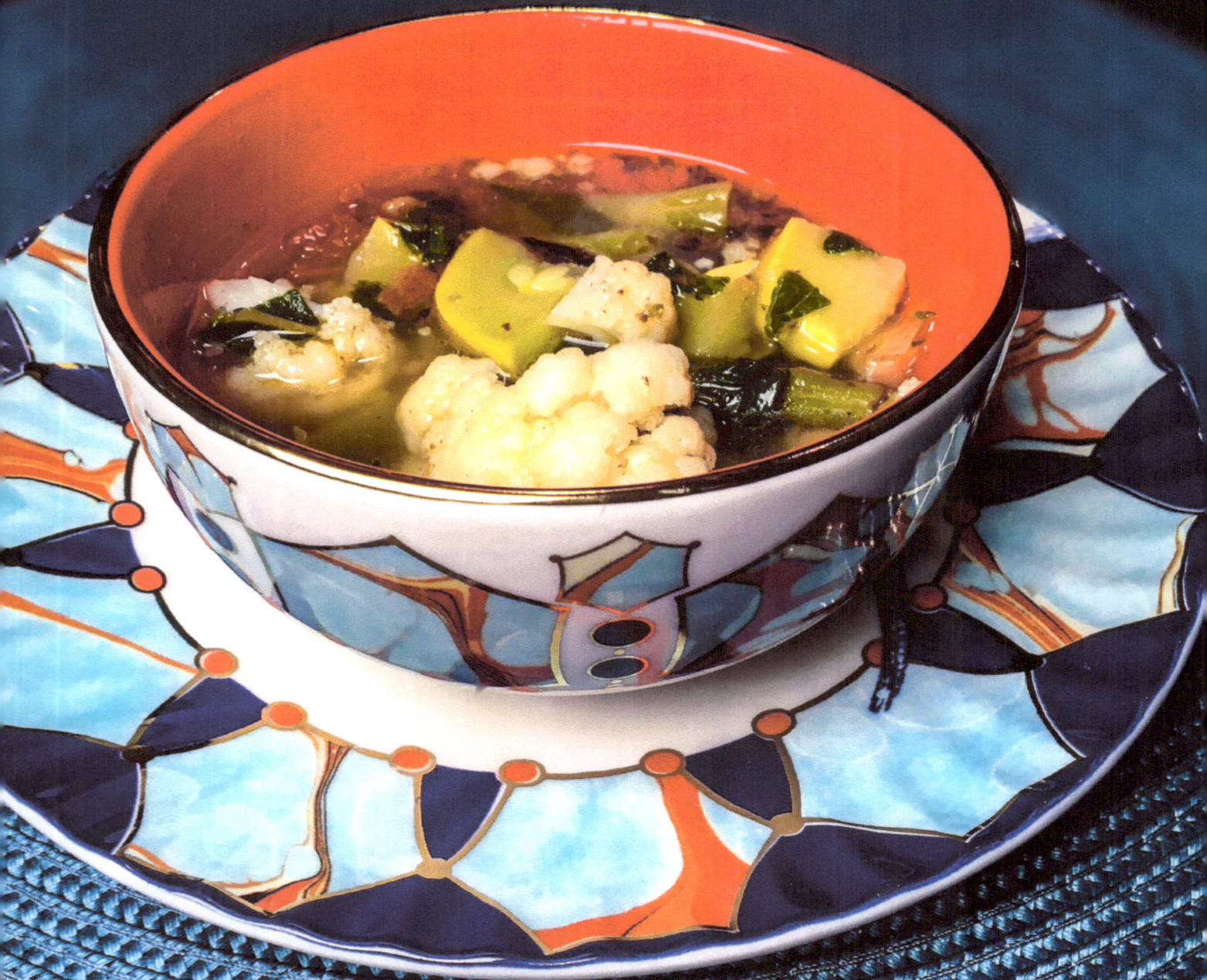

KETO KICKSTART SOUP

Okay, it's time to kickstart this diet! The Keto Kickstart Soup is the best way to enjoy a nice warm winter tradition. This soup comes loaded with flavor and nutrients that's sure to get you over the first week keto hump!

SERVINGS: 7 | SERVING SIZE: 1½ CUPS

INGREDIENTS

- **4 slices bacon (cooked+chopped)**
- **¼ cup chopped white onion**
- **1 Tbsp. garlic (minced)**
- **1 Tbsp. olive oil**
- **¼ cup sun-dried tomatoes**
- **9 cups chicken stock/broth**
- **2 cups cauliflower**
- **2 cups cooked chicken breast (cubed or shredded)**
- **1 cup yellow squash, sliced**
- **1 cup green beans**
- **2 cups swiss/rainbow chard**
- **salt and pepper to taste**

STEPS

1. In a large pot, sauté the onions and cooked bacon with the olive oil on medium heat, until onions are golden brown.

2. Add garlic and sun-dried tomatoes. Cook for 5 minutes.

3. Add chicken stock/broth (7 cups - add remaining broth when warming up later), cauliflower and chicken. Simmer for 15 minutes.

4. Add the squash, green beans, and chard. Simmer for 10 minutes.

5. Add salt and pepper to taste.

6. When heating for later use, you can add chicken broth to stretch out the soup.

NUTRITION (PER SERV.): 1½ CUPS
Calories: 296; **Fat:** 12g; **Protein:** 34g; **Total Carbs:** 13g
Fiber: 4g, Net Carbs: 13g

NET CARBS = TOTAL CARBS - ½(FIBER*) - ½(SUGAR ALCOHOLS)
* if there is more than 5 grams of fiber in one serving, subtract half of it (not all of it)

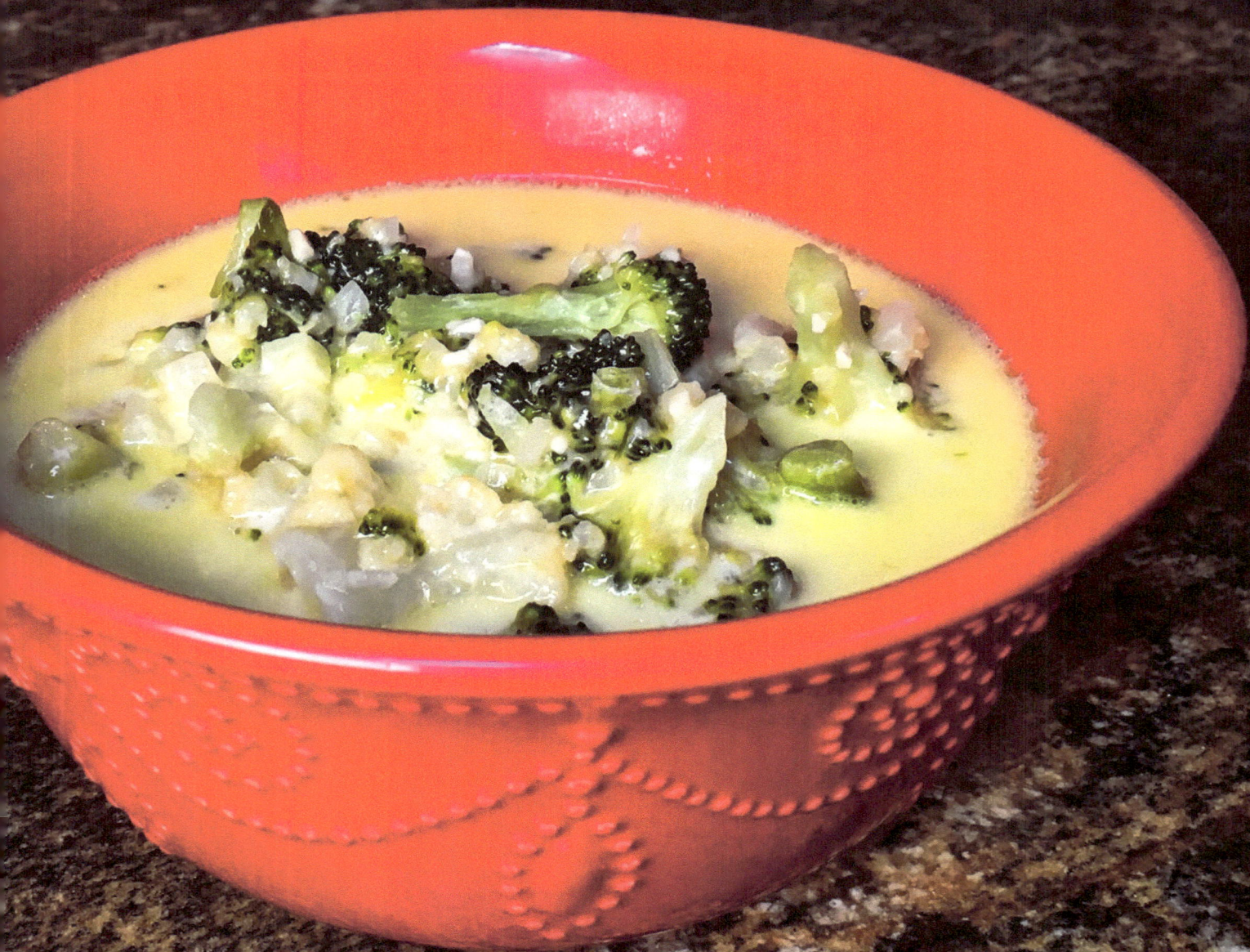

BROCCOLI CHEDDAR CAULIFLOWER SOUP

Broccoli and cheddar cheese have always been a wonderful combination, but add cream, and a bit of cauliflower and you get a creamy, full bodied soup. This popular soup is quick and easy to prepare, doesn't call for many ingredients, and the flavor is simply sublime.

SERVINGS: 7 | SERVING SIZE: 1¼ CUP

INGREDIENTS

- **2 cups broccoli florets (finely chopped)**
- **2 cups cauliflower florets (finely chopped)**
- **1 stalk celery (finely chopped)**
- **4 cup chicken stock/broth**
- **2 Tbsp. garlic (minced)**
- **1 Tbsp. olive oil**
- **1 cup heavy cream**
- **2 cups cheddar cheese (shredded)**

STEPS

1. In a large pot, sauté the garlic and celery with the olive oil on medium heat, until garlic is golden brown and celery is translucent.

2. Add chicken broth, heavy cream, broccoli, and cauliflower. Increase heat, bring to a boil, then reduce heat and simmer for 15 minutes or until broccoli and cauliflower are tender.

3. Add the shredded cheese a little at a time, stirring constantly, until cheese has melted (keep at a low simmer). Continue adding cheese until all is melted.

4. Remove from heat and serve! If you do not like chunky soup, you can run through a blender when done.

NUTRITION (PER SERV.): 1¼ CUP
Calories: 330; **Fat:** 27g; **Protein:** 13.7g; **Total Carbs:** 8g
Fiber: 2.4g, Net Carbs: 8g

NET CARBS = TOTAL CARBS - ½(FIBER*) - ½(SUGAR ALCOHOLS)
* if there is more than 5 grams of fiber in one serving, subtract half of it (not all of it)

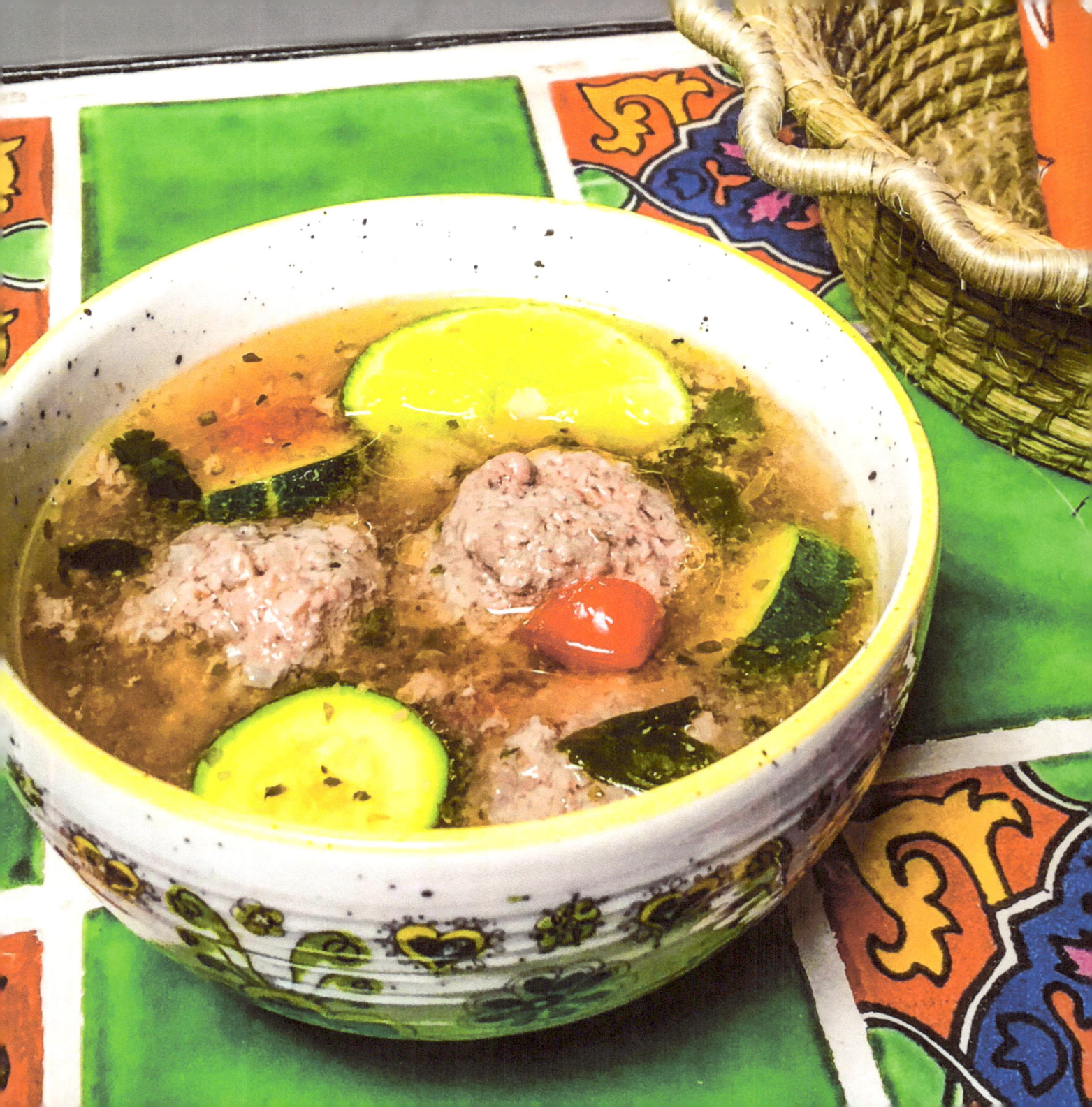

KETO ALBONDIGAS SOUP

Are you searching for that little bit of Mexican flare, are you missing the mariachi music and warm wonderful Mexican dishes? Well, do we have a soup for you... the Keto Albondigas Soup has all, if not more, of the flavor of regular Albondigas without the carbs. We take out the rice and replace it with a quilt free Mexican delight. So turn on your favorite Latin music, sit back, relax, and enjoy!

SERVINGS: 7 | SERVING SIZE: 1¼ CUP

INGREDIENTS

- 1 lb. ground beef (80/20)
- 1 egg
- 1 zucchini
- ½ cup cilantro (finely chopped)
- 2 tsp. garlic (minced)
- ½ tsp. salt
- ¼ tsp. pepper
- 1½ tsp. ground cumin
- 7 cups chicken broth
- ¼ cup white onion (diced)
- 3 stalks celery
- 1 tomato (diced)
- 1 tsp. oregano (dried)

STEPS

1. **Meatballs.** Combine ground beef, egg, 2 tsp. minced garlic, 1/4 cup cilantro, 1/2 tsp. salt, 1/4 tsp. pepper and 1 tsp. cumin. Roll meatballs between palms. Make 12-15.

2. Combine chicken broth, 1/4 cup onion, 1 tomato (diced), 3 stalks celery (chopped), 1/2 tsp. cumin, 1/4 cup cilantro, and 1 tsp. oregano in big pot.

3. Bring pot to boil, then reduce heat and simmer for 10 minutes. Bring pot to boil again and drop in meatballs to cook them. Reduce to a simmer and add sliced zucchini. Simmer 10-20 minutes until zucchini is tender.

4. Serve and enjoy this Mexican delight!

NUTRITION (PER SERV.): 1¼ CUP
Calories: 168; **Fat:** 9g; **Protein:** 18g; **Total Carbs:** 3.7g
Fiber: 0.7g, Net Carbs: 3.7g

NET CARBS = TOTAL CARBS - ½(FIBER*) - ½(SUGAR ALCOHOLS)
* if there is more than 5 grams of fiber in one serving, subtract half of it (not all of it)

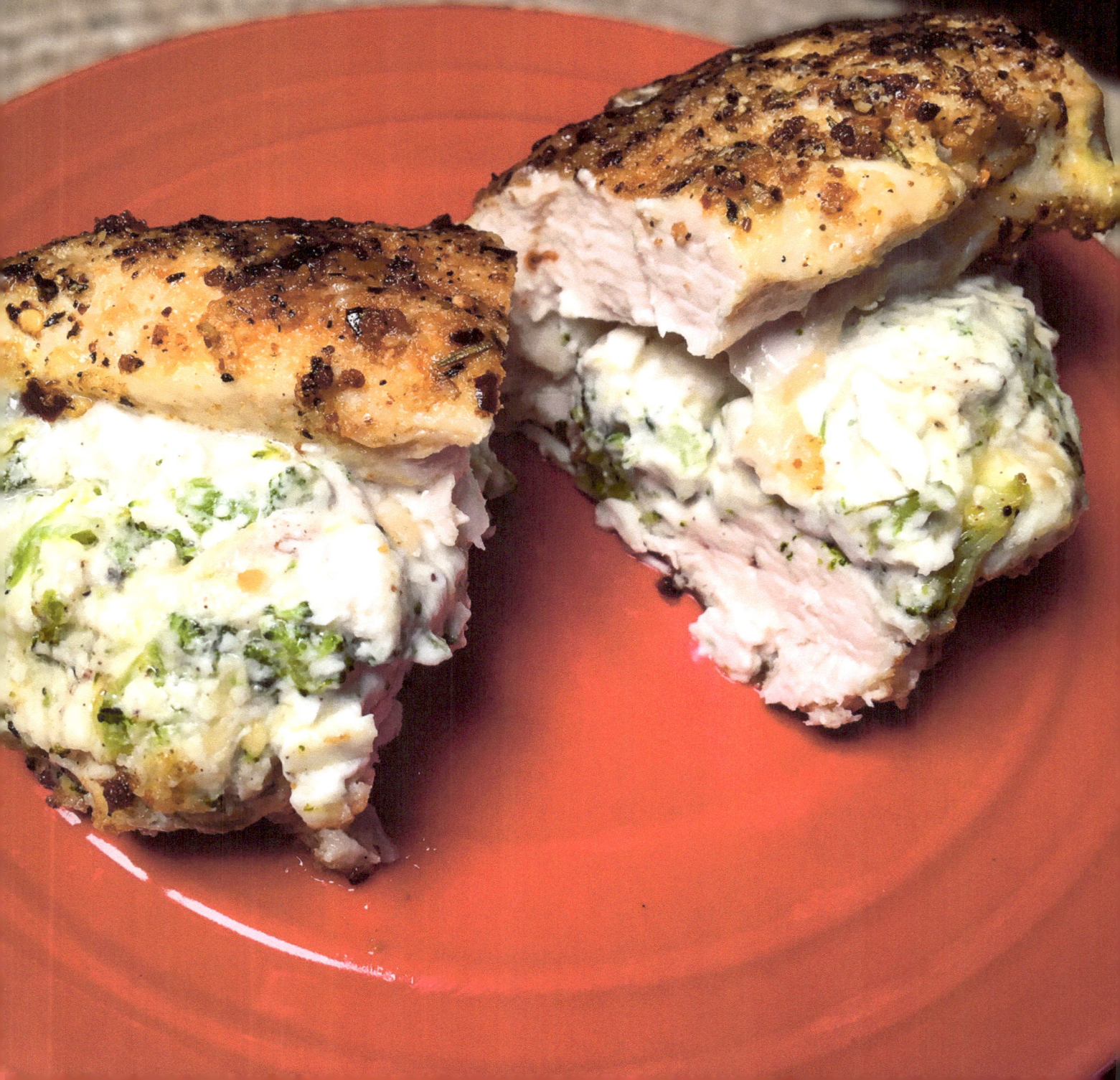

NEXT LEVEL STUFFED CHICKEN

The ultimate recipe...chicken stuffed with perfection. What is perfection you ask...cream cheese, broccoli, cheese, and a little secret ingredient.... (shhh, its cinnamon)! A pork rind and cheese crust gives this dish an ever so lovely golden crunch. Need I say more.....

SERVINGS: 8 | SERVING SIZE: ½ STUFFED CHICKEN BREAST

INGREDIENTS

- **4 large boneless chicken breasts**

STUFFING
- **6 oz. cream cheese**
- **1 cup broccoli (finely chopped)**
- **⅓ cup parmesan cheese (shredded)**
- **½ cup mozzarella cheese (shredded)**
- **½ tsp. garlic (minced)**
- **⅛ tsp. cinnamon**
- **¼ tsp. salt**
- **¼ tsp. black pepper**

BREADING
- **2 Tbsp. olive oil (for frying)**
- **2 eggs**
- **1½ cup pork rinds***
- **⅓ cup parmesan cheese (shredded)**
- **⅛ tsp. garlic powder**
- **⅛ tsp. onion powder**
- **½ tsp. salt**

STEPS

1. Preheat the oven to 375 degrees F.

2. For stuffing, combine cream cheese, garlic, parmesan, mozzarella, broccoli, cinnamon, pepper, and salt in a bowl.

3. To prepare chicken, trim off any fat, cut in half lengthwise (butterfly), then pound chicken flat with mallet (or tenderize with fork).

4. Place flattened chicken on piece of plastic wrap, spoon 1/4 of the filling mixture into the middle of the chicken cutlet and fold chicken over. (Use the plastic wrap to help fold chicken over, making sure to seal edges of chicken over the mixture). Chill the stuffed chicken for 15 minutes.

5. Repeat Steps 3 – 4 with remaining chicken breasts.

6. While chicken is chilling, prepare the breading. In a bowl combine the breading ingredients (garlic powder, onion powder, parmesan cheese, pork rinds, and salt). Whisk egg in a separate bowl.

. . . continued on next page

. . . continued

STEPS

7. Remove chicken from refrigerator and dip into beaten eggs. Lay the chicken into the breading mix and make sure to coat both sides.

8. Heat oil in a large skillet over medium-high heat. Add chicken to skillet, sear each side until golden brown.

9. Transfer chicken to baking pan. Place in oven and bake for 35-40 minutes (make sure no pink or use meat thermometer (165 deg. F)).

* *Crush pork rinds into a fine powder to best coat the chicken.*

NUTRITION (PER SERV.): ½ STUFFED CHICKEN BREAST
Calories: 342; **Fat:** 21g; **Protein:** 34.8g; **Total Carbs:** 3.5g
Fiber: 0.6g, Net Carbs: 3.5g

NET CARBS = TOTAL CARBS - ¼(FIBER*) - ¼(SUGAR ALCOHOLS)
* if there is more than 5 grams of fiber in one serving, subtract half of it (not all of it)

TASTY BONE BROTH SOUP

Move over Chicken Soup, you have officially been replaced with none other than, Bone Broth. The craze has arrived along with the wide spread knowledge of the health benefits of this nutrient dense liquid. Stores everywhere are stocked with cartons of premade bone broth making it easy to reap the benefits. Make this flavor loaded recipe anytime you need to beat a cold or sip it as a nutritious afternoon snack.

SERVINGS: 12 | SERVING SIZE: 1 CUP

INGREDIENTS

- **4 slices bacon (cooked + chopped)**
- **2 Tbsps. garlic (minced)**
- **1 celery stalk (finely chopped)**
- **2 Tbsps. olive oil**
- **8 cups bone broth (chicken)**
- **4 cups chicken stock/broth**
- **1 Tbsp. dried onions**
- **2 Tbsps. Italian Seasonings**
- **1 tsp. Salt**
- **Add any other desired seasonings**

STEPS

1. In a large pot, heat olive oil on medium-high heat, sauté garlic and cooked bacon, until garlic is golden brown.

2. Add celery. Cook for 5 minutes.

3. Add all broth and seasonings. Simmer for 15 minutes.

4. Add salt and pepper to taste.

NUTRITION (PER SERV.): 1 CUP
Calories: 62; **Fat:** 3.2g; **Protein:** 7g; **Total Carbs:** 1.3g
Fiber: 1g, Net Carbs: 1.3g

NET CARBS = TOTAL CARBS - ½(FIBER*) - ½(SUGAR ALCOHOLS)
* if there is more than 5 grams of fiber in one serving, subtract half of it (not all of it)

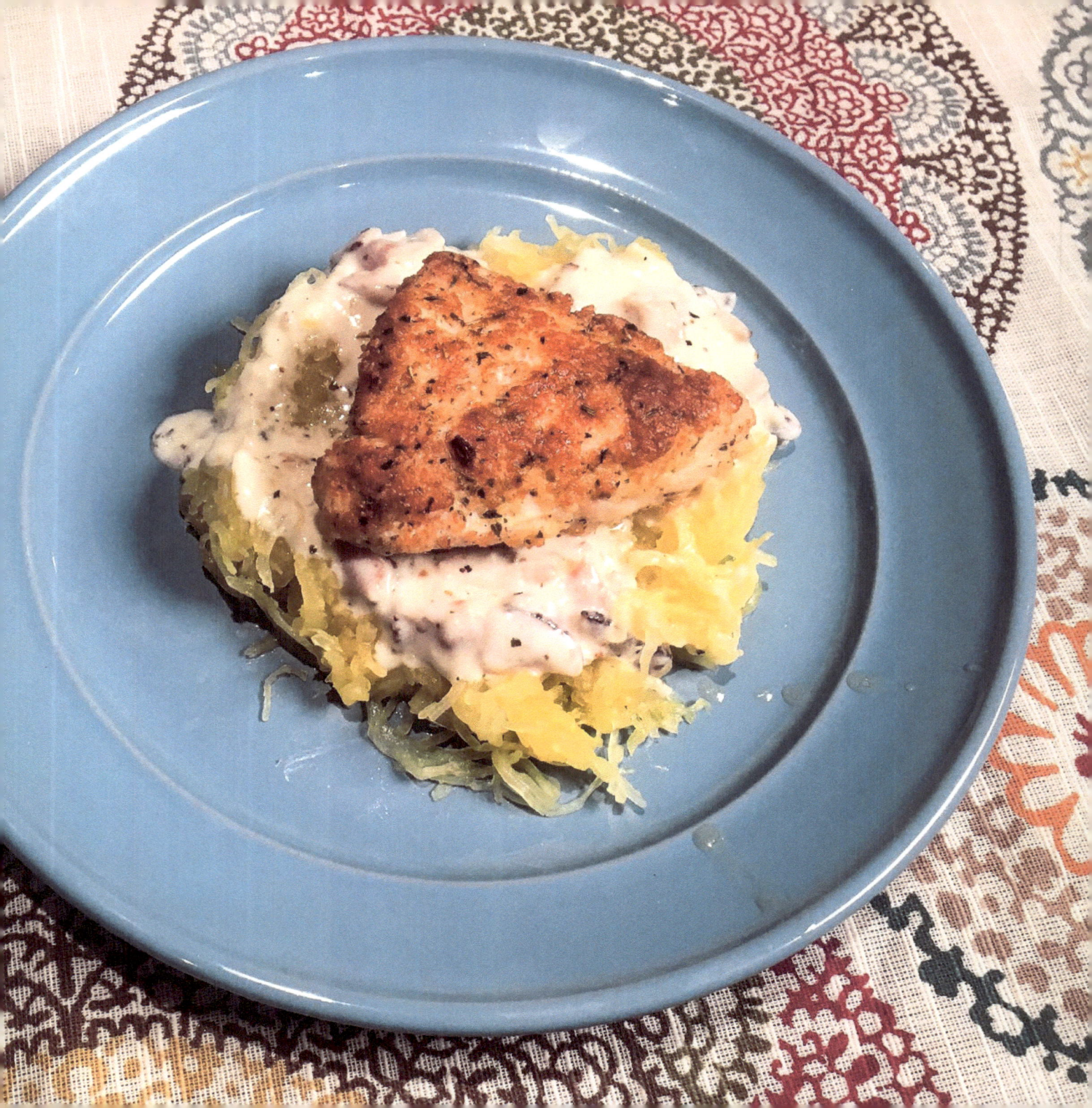

CHICKEN ALFREDO A'LA KETO

This chicken alfredo is not only keto friendly, but it's also guaranteed to be the best you've ever had! We replace the carb loaded spaghetti with none other than...spaghetti squash! Nothing against Alfredo di Lelio (the creator of alfredo sauce), but we thought we could do better, so we did, we added bacon, to give you an Italian keto delight!

SERVINGS: 8 | SERVING SIZE: ½ CHICKEN BREAST, ½ CUP SPAGHETTI SQUASH, ¼ CUP SAUCE

INGREDIENTS

- 1 Large spaghetti squash

ALFREDO SAUCE

- 1 tsp. Italian seasonings
- 1 tsp. garlic (minced)
- 1 cup heavy cream
- ¼ cup butter
- 1½ cups parmesan cheese
- 4 bacon slices (crumbled)
- ¼ cup chicken broth

CHICKEN + BREADING

- 4 boneless chicken breasts
- 2 Tbsps. olive oil (for frying)
- 1 eggs
- ⅔ cup parmesan cheese (grated)
- ¼ tsp. onion powder
- 1 tsp. Italian seasonings
- 1 tsp. salt

STEPS

1. **Spaghetti Squash.** Puncture with a fork/knife (several times) and microwave 20-30 min. (depending on size of squash), flip over halfway through (squash is done once sides are soft). Cut in half once done. Scrape out seeds, then scrape out spaghetti flesh with a fork. (Caution: HOT)

2. **Chicken + Breading.** Beat the eggs in a medium bowl. Combine breading ingredients in separate bowl. Heat the oil in a medium pan. Cut chicken in half then dip into egg, then breading mix. In pan, heat olive oil and brown chicken on both sides, then transfer chicken to baking pan. Bake for 35-40 minutes at 375 degrees F (make sure no pink).

3. **Alfredo Sauce.** Melt butter in saucepan on medium low heat. Add cream and chicken broth, simmer for 5 minutes. Add garlic, cheese, Italian seasonings, and bacon.

4. Dish ½ cup spaghetti squash onto plate, add ½ chicken breast, top off with 1/4 cup alfredo sauce. Now enjoy!

NUTRITION (PER SERV.): SEE ABOVE
Calories: 457; **Fat:** 33g; **Protein:** 32g; **Total Carbs:** 8g
Fiber: 0.8g, Net Carbs: 8g

NET CARBS = TOTAL CARBS - ½(FIBER*) - ½(SUGAR ALCOHOLS)
* if there is more than 5 grams of fiber in one serving, subtract half of it (not all of it)

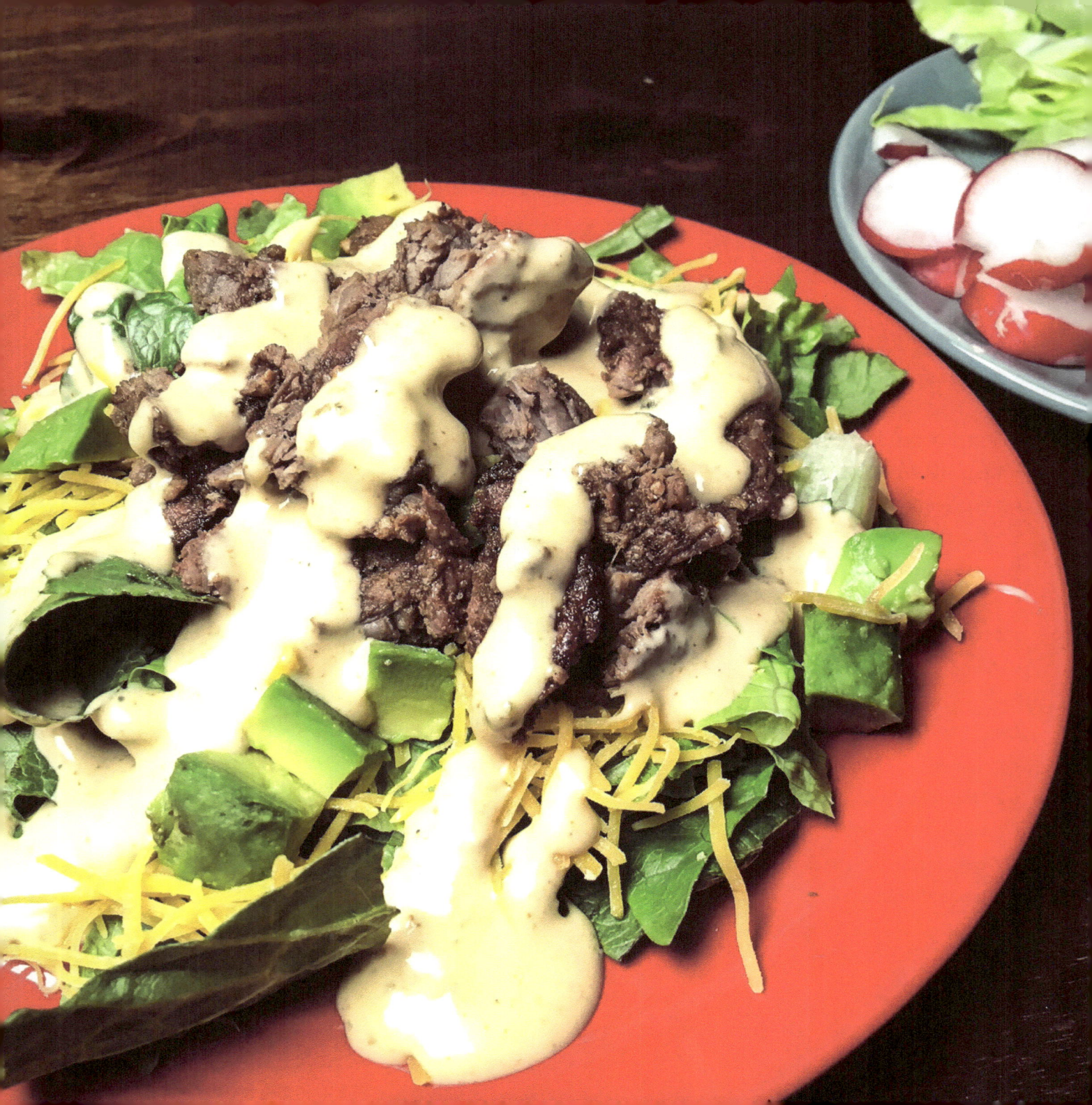

KETO TEX-MEX SALAD

It is time for some Taco Salad (hold the taco)! Taco salads are a time honored tradition among dieters and healthy-minds a-like. However, on keto, we want to kill the carbs, so here is an ever so tasty Skirt Steak Salad with all of the fixings minus the carbs.

SERVINGS: 7 | SERVING SIZE: ¼ - ½ AVOCADO, 2 CUPS LETTUCE, ¼ CUP CHEESE, 2 TBSP. DRESSING, ¼ CUP MEAT

INGREDIENTS

- 1 lb. skirt steak

MARINADE

- 1 Tbsp. garlic (minced)
- ½ Tbsp. salt
- 2 tsp. pepper
- ½ cup chicken broth
- ¼ cup olive oil
- 1 tsp. onion powder
- 1 Tbsp. cilantro (chopped)
- 1 tsp. ground cumin
- 1 tsp. chili powder

SALAD

- 3 avocados (cubed)
- 1-2 bags romaine lettuce
- 1 bag cheddar cheese (shredded)
- 1 bottle chipotle salad dressing

(less than 2g carbs/serv)

STEPS

1. Season Skirt Steak. Prepare night before. Pound the meat until ¼ inch thick. In large bowl combine all marinade ingredients. The marinade will be more like a paste. Rub mixture on meat then marinade overnight in the refrigerator.

2. Cook Skirt Steak. Prepare grill and throw steak on grill. Grill on medium-high heat for 6-8 minutes, flipping midway through. Remove from heat and cut into ¼ inch cubes.

3. Combine Salad + Meat. Prepare the salad servings as needed, otherwise the lettuce will get soggy. Each serving includes:
- ¼ - ½ avocado (cubed)
- 2 cups romaine lettuce
- ¼ cup cheddar cheese (shredded)
- 2 Tbsp. chipotle style salad dressing
- ¼ cup meat (¼" cubed)

* Store salad and meat separate and dish out each day.

NUTRITION (PER SERV.): ⅟₇ OF RECIPE
Calories: 538; **Fat:** 44.5g; **Protein:** 26g; **Total Carbs:** 13g
Fiber: 9g, Net Carbs: 8.5g

NET CARBS = TOTAL CARBS - ½(FIBER*) - ½(SUGAR ALCOHOLS)
* if there is more than 5 grams of fiber in one serving, subtract half of it (not all of it)

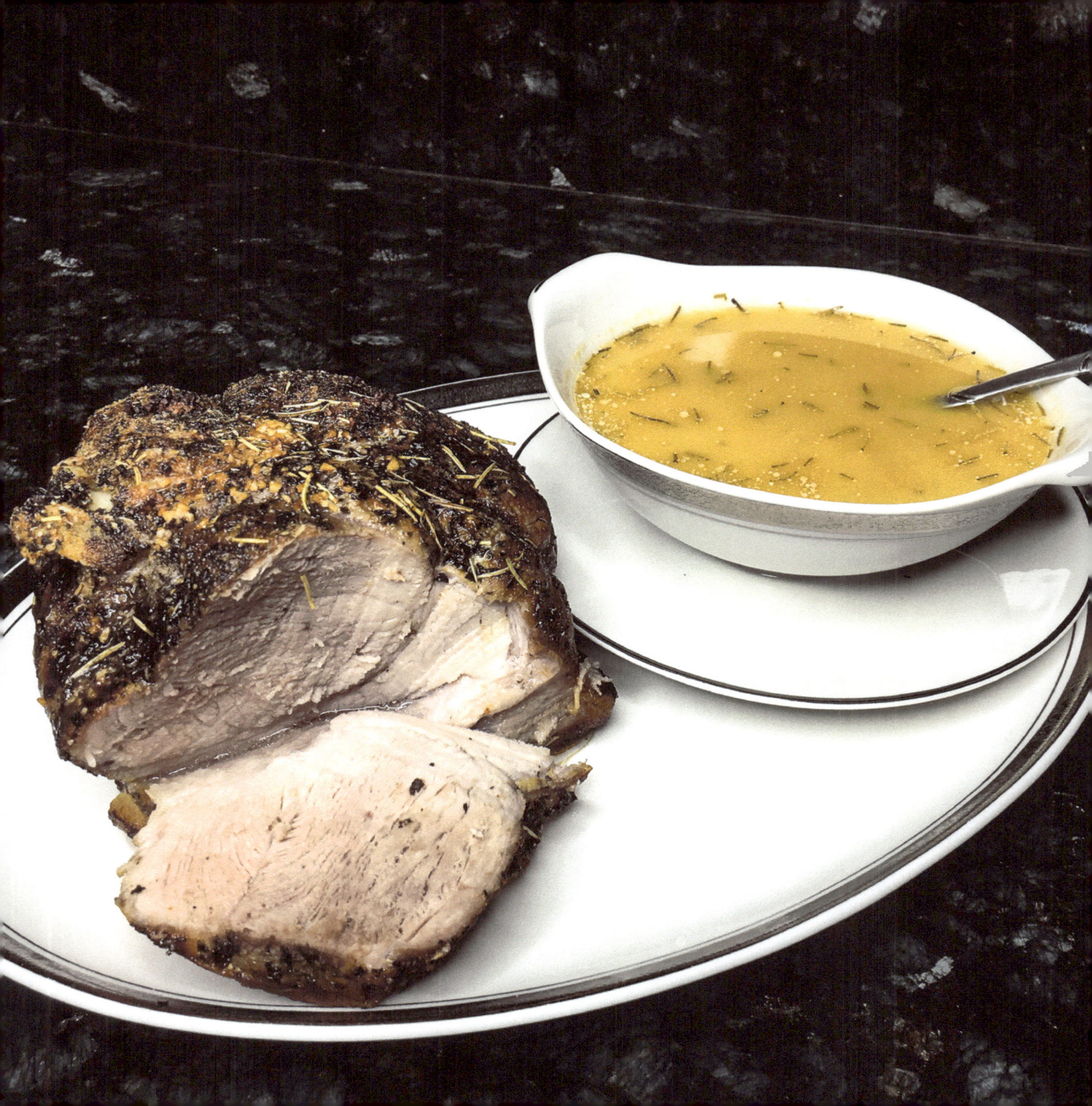

PERFECT PORK ROAST WITH KETO GRAVY

This holiday delight can now be an everyday treat! This method produces the perfect roast, a juicy and tender meat, crusted in herbs that is sure to melt in your mouth. The flavorful keto friendly gravy is a perfect accompaniment to round out this dish.

SERVINGS: 10 | SERVING SIZE: 1 CUP CUT PORK, ¼ CUP GRAVY

INGREDIENTS

PORK
- **1 Pork Shoulder Roast (boneless)**
- **4 Tbsp. olive oil**
- **2 - 4 Tbsp. garlic powder**
- **2 - 4 Tbsp. Italian Seasonings**
- **2 Tbsp. rosemary**
- **¼ tsp. black pepper**

GRAVY
- **All Pork Drippings**
- **½ - 1 cup heavy cream**

STEPS

1. Preheat oven to 325 degrees F.

2. Season pork with garlic powder, Italian seasonings, salt, pepper, and rosemary.

3. Heat 4 Tbsp. of olive oil on med-high heat. Sauté roast on all sides until brown. Transfer pork and all juices into baking dish.

4. Bake uncovered for 1 hour. Take out and pour drippings over meat. Cover pan with tin foil and return to oven for another 1½ - 2 hours (until internal pork temp reaches 175).

5. **GRAVY:** Take all drippings from pork roast and add ½ - 1 cup of heavy cream, stir in until desired consistency.

NUTRITION (PER SERV.): 1 CUP CUT PORK, ¼ CUP GRAVY
Calories: 642; Fat: 51g; Protein: 43g; Total Carbs: 2.7g
Fiber: 0.8g, Net Carbs: 2.7g

NET CARBS = TOTAL CARBS - ½(FIBER*) - ½(SUGAR ALCOHOLS)
* if there is more than 5 grams of fiber in one serving, subtract half of it (not all of it)

KETO CHICKEN SALAD

This American-classic is a perfect keto lunch or snack. Have it on its own or serve with bacon on a bed of lettuce.

SERVINGS: 4 | SERVING SIZE: ½ CUP

INGREDIENTS

- 2 - 5 oz. cans (canned Chicken Breast in water)
- 1 stalk celery (finely diced)
- 3 Tbsp. real mayonnaise
- ⅛ tsp. salt
- ⅛ tsp. pepper

STEPS

1. Combine chicken, mayonnaise, celery, salt, and pepper in a bowl.

NUTRITION (PER SERV.): ½ CUP
Calories: 128.2; **Fat:** 9g; **Protein:** 11.4g; **Total Carbs:** 0.4g
Fiber: 0.2g, Net Carbs: 0.4g

NET CARBS = TOTAL CARBS - ½(FIBER*) - ½(SUGAR ALCOHOLS)
* if there is more than 5 grams of fiber in one serving, subtract half of it (not all of it)

KETO EGG SALAD

This egg salad is sure to make an appearance at every backyard BBQ and picnic. The quick and easy recipe can be made in minutes to serve as a tasty lunch or snack. Go beyond the basics and add some low-carb relish or black olives.

SERVINGS: 2 | SERVING SIZE: 1/2 CUP

INGREDIENTS

- **4 large eggs**
- **1 stalk celery (finely diced)**
- **¹/₃ cup real mayonnaise**
- **¹/₂ tsp. mustard**
- **¹/₈ tsp. salt**
- **¹/₈ tsp. pepper**

STEPS

1. **BOIL EGGS.** Place eggs in pot large enough to hold them in a single layer. ADD cold water to cover eggs (1 inch above eggs). HEAT over high heat, bringing water to rolling boil. REMOVE from heat and cover pot with lid, let cook for 15 minutes. REMOVE eggs and place in a bowl of ice water. Allow to cool completely, then peel and cut the eggs. (Or buy hardboiled eggs from store).

2. Combine celery, mayonnaise, mustard, eggs, salt, and pepper in a bowl.

NUTRITION (PER SERV.): ½ CUP
Calories: 402; **Fat:** 38g; **Protein:** 13g; **Total Carbs:** 2g
Fiber: 0.4g, Net Carbs: 2g

NET CARBS = TOTAL CARBS - ½(FIBER*) - ½(SUGAR ALCOHOLS)
* if there is more than 5 grams of fiber in one serving, subtract half of it (not all of it)

SIDES + SNACKS

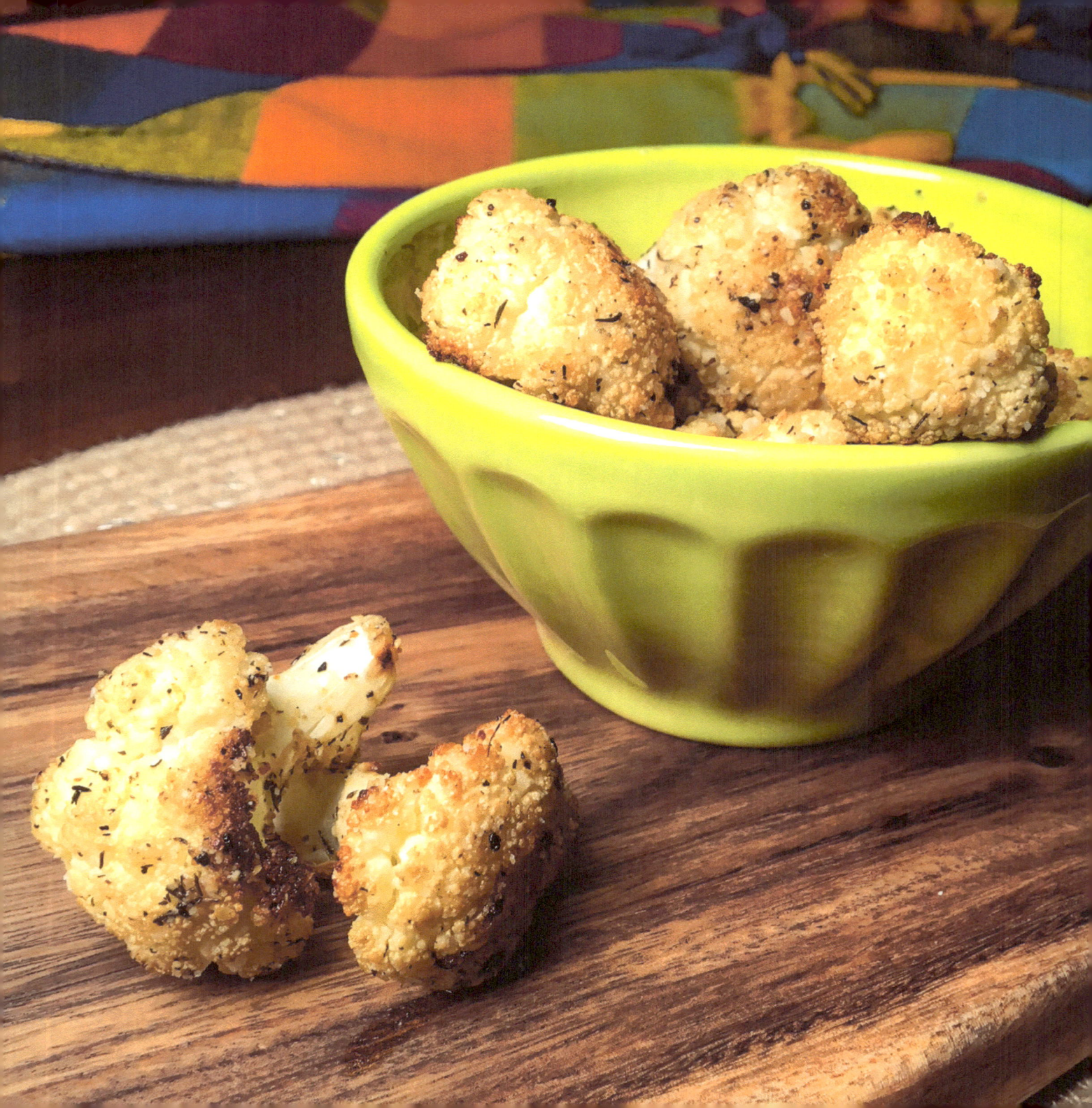

PARMESAN ROASTED CAULIFLOWER

The biggest veggie baking obsession to hit the low-carb forums! Add this perfect side dish to any meal! This side dish is sure to make you forget about those past carb experiences. Rethink your side dish without giving up on flavor.

SERVINGS: 10 - 12 | SERVING SIZE: ¼ CUP

INGREDIENTS

- 1 head cauliflower
- 1 tsp. thyme
- 1 Tbsp. garlic (minced)
- 3 Tbsps. olive oil
- ⅓ cup parmesan cheese (grated)
- ½ tsp. salt

STEPS

1. Preheat oven to 425 degrees F.

2. Cut cauliflower into florets. In a bowl add cauliflower, thyme, garlic, olive oil, and salt, toss to combine well. Place on greased cooking sheet in a single layer.

3. Roast 35-40 minutes (tossing occasionally). Add parmesan, toss to combine, then continue to roast (10-12 minutes more).

4. Remove from oven and enjoy!

NUTRITION (PER SERV.): ¼ CUP
Calories: 65; **Fat:** 4.4g; **Protein:** 2.2g; **Total Carbs:** 4.2g
Fiber: 1.4g, Net Carbs: 4.2g

NET CARBS = TOTAL CARBS - ½(FIBER*) - ½(SUGAR ALCOHOLS)
* if there is more than 5 grams of fiber in one serving, subtract half of it (not all of it)

PARMESAN ROASTED GREEN BEANS

Parmesan Roasted Green Beans are a great way to get in your veggies! Enjoy this crispy and cheesy coated dish as a side dish or snack. Minimal ingredients, extraordinary results.

SERVINGS: 4 | SERVING SIZE: ½ CUP CUT

INGREDIENTS

- **12 oz. green beans**
- **½ tsp. garlic powder**
- **2 Tbsps. olive oil**
- **2 Tbsps. garlic (miced)**
- **⅓ cup parmesan cheese (grated)**
- **½ tsp. salt**

STEPS

1. Preheat oven to 425 degrees F.

2. In a bowl combine the garlic powder, minced garlic, olive oil, and salt together.

3. Add in green beans and coat well.

4. Add parmesan, toss to combine, spread out on greased baking sheet.

5. Bake for 15 minutes or until crispy.

6. Remove from oven and enjoy!

NUTRITION (PER SERV.): ½ CUP CUT
Calories: 128; **Fat:** 9.3g; **Protein:** 4.1g; **Total Carbs:** 7g
Fiber: 3g, Net Carbs: 7g

NET CARBS = TOTAL CARBS - ½(FIBER*) - ½(SUGAR ALCOHOLS)
* if there is more than 5 grams of fiber in one serving, subtract half of it (not all of it)

OVEN ROASTED ASPARAGUS

Asparagus is packed with good for you vitamins and minerals like vitamin A, C, E, and K, as well as iron, calcium, and lots of fiber. Thanks to all the nutrients, asparagus is a good low-carb veggie option for keto goers looking for a tasty side dish.

SERVINGS: 4 | SERVING SIZE: ½ CUP CUT

INGREDIENTS

- 3 Tbsps. olive oil
- 1 bunch asparagus
- 2 Tbsps. minced garlic
- salt and pepper to taste

STEPS

1. Preheat oven to 425 degrees F.

2. Place asparagus into mixing bowl, drizzle with olive oil, garlic, add salt and pepper to taste.

3. Arrange on a baking sheet in a single layer.

4. Bake for 12-15 minutes or until tender.

NUTRITION (PER SERV.): ½ CUP CUT
Calories: 108; **Fat:** 10g; **Protein:** 1.3g; **Total Carbs:** 3.1g
Fiber: 1g, Net Carbs: 3.1g

NET CARBS = TOTAL CARBS - ½(FIBER*) - ½(SUGAR ALCOHOLS)
* if there is more than 5 grams of fiber in one serving, subtract half of it (not all of it)

CHEESY MASHED CAULIFLOWER

The ultimate in keto comfort food! Loaded with flavor and a little kick from the pepper jack cheese, this dish is sure to make you forget about the old carb filled mashed potatoes. For a more loaded dish and an added punch you can add chives, bacon and even switch out the cheese to a sharp cheddar.

SERVINGS: 7 | SERVING SIZE: ½ CUP

INGREDIENTS

- 1 large head cauliflower
- ½ - 1 cup heavy cream
- 1 cup pepper jack cheese (or preferred) (shredded)
- 2 Tbsps. butter
- salt and pepper to taste

STEPS

1. Chop cauliflower into pieces (make sure to throw out the stem, store bought riced cauliflower is mostly the stems and is harder and tasteless). Place cauliflower in large pot and cover with water. Bring to boil, then reduce to a simmer until cauliflower is tender.

2. Drain cauliflower, mash, then add butter and ½ -1 cup heavy cream, (whip until desired consistency).

3. Mix in 1 cup pepper jack cheese and add salt and pepper as desired.

NUTRITION (PER SERV.): ½ CUP
Calories: 123; **Fat:** 10.2g; **Protein:** 4.8g; **Total Carbs:** 3g
Fiber: 1.6g, Net Carbs: 3g

NET CARBS = TOTAL CARBS - ½(FIBER*) - ½ (SUGAR ALCOHOLS)
* if there is more than 5 grams of fiber in one serving, subtract half of it (not all of it)

GREEN SALAD W/ RANCH

SERVINGS: 1

INGREDIENTS

- 1 cup green salad mix (or spinach)
- 1 Tbsp. parmesan cheese (grated/shredded)
- 1 Tbsp. ranch dressing
- 1 slice bacon (crumbled)
- pepper + salt to taste

STEPS

1. Combine all ingredients and enjoy!

NUTRITION (PER SERV.): 1 SERVING
Calories: 156; **Fat:** 13g; **Protein:** 7g; **Total Carbs:** 2.7g
Fiber: 0.7g, Net Carbs: 2.7g

NET CARBS = TOTAL CARBS - ½(FIBER*) - ½(SUGAR ALCOHOLS)
* if there is more than 5 grams of fiber in one serving, subtract half of it (not all of it)

GREEN SALAD W/ OLIVE OIL + CUCUMBERS

SERVINGS: 1

INGREDIENTS

- 1 cup green salad mix (or spinach)
- 2 cucumber slices
- 1 Tbsp. parmesan cheese (grated/shredded)
- 1 Tbsp. olive oil
- 1 slice bacon (crumbled)
- pepper + salt to taste

STEPS

1. Combine all ingredients and enjoy!

NUTRITION (PER SERV.): 1 SERVING
Calories: 208; **Fat:** 19.6g; **Protein:** 7g; **Total Carbs:** 1g
Fiber: 0.5g, Net Carbs: 1g

NET CARBS = TOTAL CARBS - ½(FIBER*) - ½(SUGAR ALCOHOLS)
* if there is more than 5 grams of fiber in one serving, subtract half of it (not all of it)

FRENCH ONION DIP

SERVINGS: 1

INGREDIENTS

- **16 oz. sour cream**
- **1 package french onion dip**
- **½ cup real mayonnaise**

STEPS

1. Combine all ingredients and enjoy!

NUTRITION (PER SERV.): 2 TBSP.
Calories: 84; **Fat:** 8g; **Protein:** 1g; **Total Carbs:** 2g
Fiber: 0g, Net Carbs: 2g

NET CARBS = TOTAL CARBS - ½(FIBER*) - ½(SUGAR ALCOHOLS)
* if there is more than 5 grams of fiber in one serving, subtract half of it (not all of it)

DEVILED EGGS

SERVINGS: 8 HALVES | SERVING SIZE: 1 HALF

INGREDIENTS

- **4 boiled eggs**
- **2 Tbsps. mayonnaise**
- **1 tsp. mustard**
- **salt + pepper to taste**

STEPS

1. Cut eggs in half lengthwise and carefully scoop out yolk.

2. Place yolks in bowl, add mustard, mayonnaise, salt and pepper and mash.

3. Divide mixture into egg whites.

NUTRITION (PER SERV.): 1 HALF
Calories: 58.2; **Fat:** 5g; **Protein:** 2.9g; **Total Carbs:** 0.4g
Fiber: 0.1g, Net Carbs: 0.4g

NET CARBS = TOTAL CARBS - ¼(FIBER*) - ½(SUGAR ALCOHOLS)
* if there is more than 5 grams of fiber in one serving, subtract half of it (not all of it)

KETO APPROVED SNACKS

Below is a list of easy grab and go keto approved snacks. Each item is listed with its accompanying serving size, Calories, Fat, Protein, and Carbs. broken down into: Total Carbs., Fiber, and Net Carbs. The guidelines derived from the ADA and the FDA on how to calculate the amount of digestible carbs. (Net Carbs.) is given below. Recall that there are some hidden carbs. in Fiber as well as Sugar Alcohol, so follow the Net Carbs. calculation in this book (pg. 13) for a more accurate carb count. Hidden carbs. can keep you from losing weight, so be diligent.

- **FIBER:** *if the quantity of Fiber in a food is more than 5 grams (per serving), subtract half of the grams of Fiber from the Total Carbs. (not all of it).*

- **SUGAR ALCOHOL:** *if there is Sugar Alcohol in a food, subtract ½ of it from the Total Carbs. (not all of it).*

FOOD	CALORIES	FAT (g)	PROTEIN (g)	CARBS (g) (Total, Fiber, Net)
¼ Cup Walnuts	176	16.3	3.8	T: 3.4g, F: 1.7g, N: 3.4g
12 Almonds	92	7.4	3.1	T: 3.2g, F: 1.8g, N: 3.2g
1 Deviled Egg Half	58	5	2.9	T: 0.4g, F: 0.1g, N: 0.4g
1 String Cheese	82	6	7	T: 0g, F:0 g, N: 0g
1 Sugar Free Jell-O Cup	10*	0	1	T: 0g, F: 0g, N: 0g
12 Almonds + 1 String Cheese	174	13.4	10.1	T: 3.2g, F: 1.8g, N: 3.2g
¼ Cup Sliced Cucumber + 2 Tbsp. French Onion Dip	89	8	1.2	T: 3g, F: 0.3g, N: 3g
3 Pepperoni Slices + 3 (½" Cubes) Cheese	22	2	1	T: 0g, F: 0g, N: 0g
Celery Stick + 1 Laughing Cow Cheese Wedge	32	1.6	2.3	T: 2.2g, F: 0.6g, N: 2.2g

* Nutrition Labels are not always accurate, the FDA allows for a margin of error of up to 20% for the stated values vs. the actual values. Therefore, the nutrition label on a 100 calorie snack pack could be as much as 120 calories. So look at the nutrition label and be aware when things do not add up. Like in the Sugar Free Jell-O Cup above, the label calculates to be 4 calories (the only apparent calories coming from the 1 gram (4 calories of protein), not 10 calories as it states, so those extra calories are coming from somewhere.

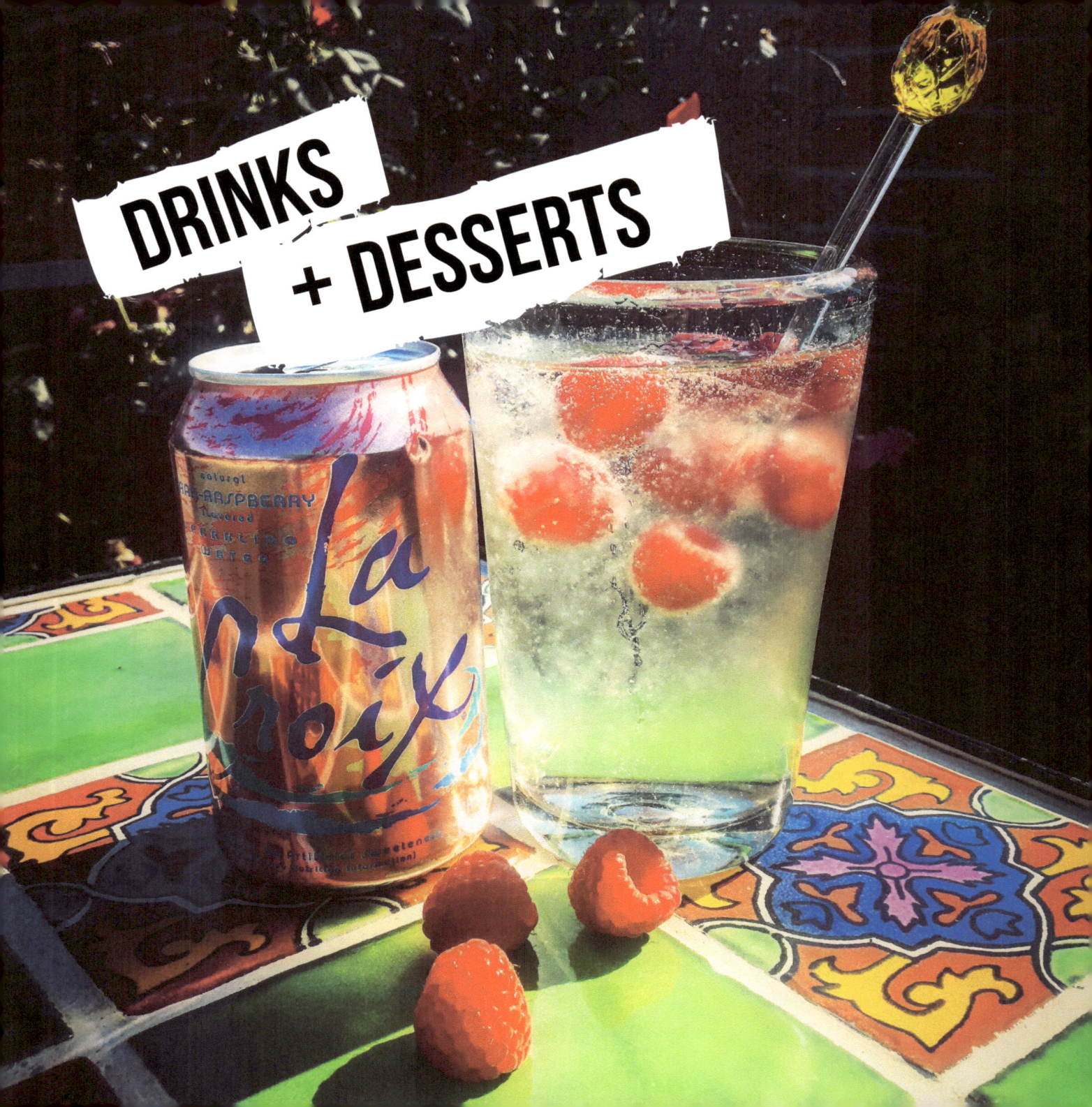

DRINKS + DESSERTS

LEMON WATER
WITH CAYENNE PEPPER
YOUR MORNING
DETOX DRINK

Start each morning with your lemon juice and cayenne pepper in warm water. Lemons are helpful in liver detoxification and they contain high amounts of vitamin C and other antioxidants. Adding the cayenne pepper can aid in lowering blood glucose levels and speed up metabolism.

SERVINGS: 1 | SERVING SIZE: 1 CUP

INGREDIENTS

- 1 cup (or 1 mug) water
- 1 - 2 Tbsp. Real Lemon Juice
- dash of cayenne pepper (enough to be hot, but not too much you can't stand it)

STEPS

1. Heat water in microwave (or cold is fine too).
2. Add lemon juice and cayenne pepper (or chili pepper).
3. Stir and enjoy with a straw (helps with acidity on teeth).

NOTE: For more of a lemonade drink, you can add a small amount of Liquid Stevia to make it sweeter (Caution: Stevia is a concentrated sweetner, very little is needed). If you add the Stevia, add more water so as to dilute the drink or it will be too sweet. Add ice to finish it off.

NUTRITION (PER SERV.): 1 CUP
Calories: 3.6; **Fat:** 0g; **Protein:** 0.1g; **Total Carbs:** 0.8g
Fiber: 0.1g, Net Carbs: 0.8g

NET CARBS = TOTAL CARBS - ½(FIBER*) - ½(SUGAR ALCOHOLS)
* if there is more than 5 grams of fiber in one serving, subtract half of it (not all of it)

KETO VANILLA FRAPPUCCINO

Those sugar filled coffee shop drinks sure are tasty, but they tend to cost a small fortune and will definitely add on the pounds. So cut out the sugar and stop wasting the money, make your favorite coffee shop drink at home. This Keto Vanilla Frappuccino is sure to impress with its smooth and creamy base accented with a touch of vanilla and cinnamon.

SERVINGS: 1

INGREDIENTS

- **1 cup unsweetened almond milk (vanilla)**
- **2 Tbsps. heavy cream**
- **$\frac{1}{8}$ cup kefir**
- **$\frac{1}{4}$ Tbsp. cinnamon (or desired amount)**
- **1 tsp. vanilla extract**
- **pinch Himalayan salt**
- **2-3 ice cubes (desired amount)**

STEPS

1. Combine all ingredients in blender and enjoy!

NUTRITION (PER SERV.): 1 CUP
Calories: 160; **Fat:** 14.5g; **Protein:** 3.3g; **Total Carbs:** 4g
Fiber: 1g, Net Carbs: 4g

NET CARBS = TOTAL CARBS - ½(FIBER*) - ½(SUGAR ALCOHOLS)
* if there is more than 5 grams of fiber in one serving, subtract half of it (not all of it)

KETO GOLD MILK

This traditional Indian beverage combines the health benefits of turmeric, black pepper, and other herbs and spices. The health benefits of golden milk are linked to the turmeric and its active ingredient, curcumin. The addition of black pepper helps boost the effects of the curcumin. This warm, healing beverage is full of natural anti-inflammatory, anti-cancer, and antioxidant ingredients.

SERVINGS: 1

INGREDIENTS

- 1 cup unsweetened almond milk (vanilla)
- ¼ cup kefir
- ¾ tsp. turmeric/curcumin powder (or 1-2 capsule broken open)
- ½ tsp. ginger powder
- ¼ tsp. cinnamon
- ¼ tsp. vanilla extract
- pinch Himalayan salt + black pepper
- 2-3 ice cubes (desired amount)

STEPS

1. Combine all ingredients in a blender and enjoy!

NUTRITION (PER SERV.): 1 CUP
Calories: 73; **Fat:** 4.8g; **Protein:** 3.5g; **Total Carbs:** 4g
Fiber: 1g, Net Carbs: 4g

NET CARBS = TOTAL CARBS - ½(FIBER*) - ½(SUGAR ALCOHOLS)
* if there is more than 5 grams of fiber in one serving, subtract half of it (not all of it)

KETO COFFEE

This jolt of caffeine and cream in the morning will energize you and keep you full for hours! If you still need some sweetness in your morning pick-me-up, you can add some cinnamon to your coffee before you brew or add a drop of your favorite flavored Liquid Stevia. If you're not one of the caffeine addicted and would like a less energetic way to start the day, you can always substitute with decaf coffee.

SERVINGS: 1

INGREDIENTS

- **1 cup unsweetened coffee**
- **1 Tbsp. heavy cream**

STEPS

1. Make 1 cup (or desired amount) of black coffee, then add 1 Tbsp. heavy cream. Enjoy the jolt of caffeine!

NUTRITION (PER SERV.): 1 CUP
Calories: 56; **Fat:** 5.5g; **Protein:** 0.7g; **Total Carbs:** 1g
Fiber: 0g, Net Carbs: 1g

NET CARBS = TOTAL CARBS - ½(FIBER*) - ½(SUGAR ALCOHOLS)
* if there is more than 5 grams of fiber in one serving, subtract half of it (not all of it)

KETO COFFEE BULLETPROOF STYLE

You can barely get a keto convo in without hearing about the infamous Keto BulletProof Coffee. Why add butter and MCT (Medium Chain Triglyceride) oil to your coffee? Well first and foremost the amount of fat that you get from this concoction is hard to beat, plus it has little to no carbs., making it a good addition to any keto morning. If you're using MCT oil it is wise to start off with a small amount, less than a teaspoon, then work your way up (some people have noted stomach problems when adding too much MCT oil). If you are more of a traditionalist, you can always substitute the Keto BulletProof Coffee with plain coffee and cream.

SERVINGS: 1

INGREDIENTS

- **1 cup unsweetened coffee**
- **2 Tbsps. unsalted butter**
- **1 Tbsp. MCT oil or coconut oil**

STEPS

1. Combine all ingredients in a blender and enjoy!

NUTRITION (PER SERV.): 1 CUP
Calories: 340g; **Fat:** 37g; **Protein:** 0.5g; **Total Carbs:** 1.1g
Fiber: 1.1g, Net Carbs: 1.1g

NET CARBS = TOTAL CARBS - ½(FIBER*) - ½(SUGAR ALCOHOLS)
* if there is more than 5 grams of fiber in one serving, subtract half of it (not all of it)

PEANUT BUTTER BONBONS

SERVINGS: 3 | SERVING SIZE: 1 BONBON

INGREDIENTS

- 1 Tbsp. creamy peanut butter
- ¼ oz. (1 Piece) Bakers Unsweetened Chocolate
- 1-2 drops Liquid Stevia
- dash of sea salt

STEPS

1. Use a teaspoon to roll peanut butter into 3 balls. Freeze for 10 minutes.

2. Melt chocolate in microwave at 30 sec. intervals until melted. Add Stevia drops for desired sweetness.

3. Coat chilled peanut butter balls in melted chocolate. Sprinkle on sea salt for an added flavor combination. Return to freezer for 20 minutes.

NUTRITION (PER SERV.): 1 BONBON
Calories: 48; **Fat:** 3.8g, **Protein:** 1.5g; **Total Carbs:** 2g
Fiber: 0.8g, Net Carbs: 2g

STRAWBERRY CHEESECAKE FATBOMBS

SERVINGS: 6 | SERVING SIZE: 1 CUBE

INGREDIENTS

- ¼ cup strawberries (sliced)
- 1 strawberry sliced
- 8 oz. cream cheese
- 1 - 3 drops Liquid Stevia

STEPS

1. Place strawberries in blender, add cream cheese and sweeten as desired with Liquid Stevia drops. Blend until smooth (may blend by hand or use beaters).

2. Place one strawberry slice at the bottom of each ice cube well (use silicone trey). Pour mixture over top.

3. Freeze for a tasty keto dessert.

NUTRITION (PER SERV.): 1/6 OF RECIPE
Calories: 137; **Fat:** 13g; **Protein:** 2.4g; **Total Carbs:** 2.6g
Fiber: 0.1g, Net Carbs: 2.6g

ALMOND JOY FATBOMBS

SERVINGS: 3 | SERVING SIZE: 1 PIECE

INGREDIENTS

- 3 Tbsps. unsweetened coconut flakes
- ½ oz. (2 Pieces) Bakers Unsweetened Chocolate
- 1-2 drops Liquid Stevia
- 2 Tbsps. coconut oil

STEPS

1. Mix coconut flakes with coconut oil, then form into 3 balls. Place 1 almond on each ball then freeze 10 minutes.

2. Melt chocolate in microwave at 30 sec. intervals until melted. Add Stevia drops for desired sweetness.

3. Coat chilled cononut ball in melted chocolate. Return to freezer for 20 minutes.

NUTRITION (PER SERV.): 1 PIECE
Calories: 145; **Fat:** 14.6g, **Protein:** 1g; **Total Carbs:** 2.5g
Fiber: 1.8g, Net Carbs: 2.5g

CHOCOLATE COATED WALNUTS

SERVINGS: 1 | SERVING SIZE: ¼ CUP

INGREDIENTS

- ¼ oz. (1 Piece) Bakers Unsweetened Chocolate
- 1 drop Liquid Stevia
- ¼ cup walnut halves
- dash of sea salt

STEPS

1. Melt chocolate in microwave at 30 sec. intervals until melted. Add Stevia drops for desired sweetness.

2. Coat the walnuts or drizzle with melted chocolate.

3. Sprinkle on sea salt for an added flavor combination.

NUTRITION (PER SERV.): ¼ CUP
Calories: 219; **Fat:** 19.8g; **Protein:** 4.8g; **Total Carbs:** 5.4g
Fiber: 3.2g, Net Carbs: 5.4g

EXTRA
EXTRA

YOU GET IT ALL WITH THIS MEAL PLAN

You didn't think that was it did you? We have lots of fun goodies we developed as useful resources for your hectic life. With the KT 28-Day Meal Plan you get it all; you get the meal plans, grocery lists, recipes and more...

There is a **Table of Equivalents** to help you with any conversion issues you may have. There is an **Eating Out Guide** to aid in decision making if you find yourself out to dinner with family or friends while on keto.

If you have goals, which ...you know you do, it's time to record and track those goals. Use the **Goal Tracker** and Body Measurement Guide at the back of this book to track your progress. This meal plan was designed in conjunction with **The CONCEPT24® Planner**, a wonderful resource that will help you keep track of the rest of your life while helping you get the body you deserve!

For additional information on recipes, workouts and more:

VISIT WWW.DRAEKK.COM

TABLE OF EQUIVALENTS

LIQUID/DRY MEASUREMENTS

U.S.	METRIC
¼ tsp.	1.25 mL
½ tsp.	2.5 mL
1 tsp.	5 mL
1 Tbsp. (3 tsp.)	15 mL
1 fluid oz. (2 Tbsps.)	30 mL
¼ cup	60 mL
½ cup	120 mL
1 cup	240 mL
1 pint (2 cups)	480 mL
1 quart (4 cups)	960 mL
1 gallon (16 cups)	3.8 L
1 oz. (by weight)	28 g
1 lb.	448 g
2.2 lbs	1 kg

OVEN TEMPERATURES

FAHRENHEIT (°F)	CELCIUS (°C)
300	150
325	160
350	180
375	190
400	200
425	220
450	230
475	240

LENGTHS

U.S.	METRIC
⅛ inch.	3 mm
¼ inch.	6 mm
½ inch.	12 mm
1 inch.	2.5 cm

Exact measurements have been rounded for your convenience.

TOP TIPS FOR EATING OUT ON A KETO/LOW-CARB DIET

Eating out doesn't mean you have to break your keto or low-carb lifestyle! Follow these tips and strategies and you will be able to enjoy a dinner out without the guilt.

1. DO YOUR RESEARCH

Before you go out to eat, look up the menu online (if available). There is no shame in examining a menu to see if there is anything you can eat, or even want to eat there. Take pride in knowing you have ownership over your meals!

2. SKIP THE PRE-DINNER BREAD OR CHIPS

This is really a diet saver and you will not have to exercise your willpower. Tell the waiter to not bring the bread or chips. If you are very hungry or feel cheated from missing those tasty yet empty carbs, order a low-carb appetizer instead.

3. THE ART OF SELF PORTIONING

Today's Super-Sized mindset at restaurants have distorted our view on healthy portion sizes. We sit down to dinner and expect huge portions that fill our even larger dinner plate. In the last 20 years portion sizes have doubled and even tripled in some cases. Here are some strategies to ensure you will have an enjoyable meal out without the guilt of overeating.

- **ORDER AN APPETIZER – AS YOUR MAIN MEAL**. Appetizer portion sizes are usually smaller than the main entrees, this is a good way of portion sizing. It is usually cheaper than an entree too! Win win!

- **BOX HALF YOUR FOOD ORDER.** Upon ordering, ask the waiter to box up half of your order, tell them you want to take it home. That way you will get half of the meal (which is closer to the portion size that people SHOULD eat). The bonus is you get two meals for one, also a money saver!

- **PORTION SIZE RULE OF THUMB.** Use a visual queue – use your hand to determine your portion sizes:

  - Meat – use your PALM to determine the portion size of meat (place your flat hand palm side up near the meat, the meat should be the size of just your palm).

  - Vegetables – use your FIST to determine your portion of vegetables (make a fist and see if your veggies are in a pile the same size as your FIST).

- **ORDER ALL SAUCES AND SALAD DRESSINGS ON THE SIDE.** Sauces and salad dressings at restaurants are usually full of sugar, so ordering them on the side is the best way of controlling how much you use.

4. ALL YOU CAN EAT BUFFET

ONLY use the smaller plate to get your food, you are less likely to overeat if you fill up the smaller plate (even if you go back up multiple times – use the small plate). This is also a good rule of thumb for at-home dinners, start using the smaller side plates, it's portion sizing without having to think.

FOOD FOR THOUGHT
Examples on What to Eat Out While On A Keto/Low-Carb Diet

AMERICAN FOOD / STEAK HOUSE
- Burger with No Bun
- Steak of Any Kind (High Fat Okay)
- Chicken Sandwich (No Bun)
- Chicken
- Salmon
- Cheese - Most cheeses are low-carb. (Stay clear of ricotta and cottage cheese as they are higher in carbs.)
- Butter
- Cauliflower
- Broccoli
- Carrots (make sure to use the FIST portion size guide)
- Green Beans (make sure to use the FIST portion size guide)
- Salad (NO croutons or candied nuts)
- Salad Dressings (order on the side)
- Dressings: Ranch, Caesar, Blue Cheese, Olive Oil/Vinegar (No Italian Dressing)

If you are on a Keto/Low-Carb Diet, Italian and Mexican restaurants are not advisable, but if you have a special meal planned at an Italian or Mexican restaurant try the low-carb options listed below.

ITALIAN
- Antipasti – Salami, Pastrami, Olives, Cheeses
- Caprese Salad
- Caesar Salad (No croutons)

MEXICAN
- Guacamole (eat with a spoon)
- Salsa (eat with a spoon)
- Tostada (Do Not Eat the Shell)
- Fajitas, Shredded Chicken, Carnitas, Carne Asada (Any Meats)
- Taco Salad (No Rice or Beans)

CONDIMENTS
Most sauces and traditional seasonings have added sugars and are not low-carb or keto friendly.
- ALLOWED: Yellow Mustard, Mayonnaise, Horseradish, Worcestershire Sauce

BOTTOM LINE
DO NOT mix your carbs. and fats. Eat out sparingly on keto, it is so easy to get kicked out of ketosis because of all of the hidden carbs.

TRACK YOUR PROGRESS

Remember to strive for progress, not perfection! Use the space on the opposite page to track the progress of your physical features. If the pounds are not falling off, you can still see your progress with measurements. It is best to have another person take your measurements for you, however, if you are a DIY'er, follow the guide below. Always use the same measuring tape or device to ensure accuracy. Do not obsess over the numbers, every little 1/100th of an inch is progress in the right direction!

BODY MEASUREMENT GUIDE

% BODY FAT: There are numerous ways to measure Body Fat %: Skin Calipers, Bioelectrical Impedance, Hydrostatic Weighing, 3D Body Scans, etc.

UPPER ARM: Stand erect with arms hanging freely at sides, hands facing thighs, a horizontal measurement is taken 4 inches above the elbow.

FOREARM: Stand erect with arms hanging at sides, slightly away from the body. Take a horizontal measurement at the widest circumference.

WAIST: Stand erect, arms at sides, feet together, and stomach relaxed. Take a horizontal measurement at the narrowest part of the torso (just above the belly button).

BUTTOCKS / HIPS: Standing erect, feet slightly apart (8 inches), take a horizontal measurement at maximum circumference of the buttocks.

UPPER THIGH: Standing erect, legs slightly apart (4 inches), take a horizontal measurement at the maximum circumference of the upper thigh, just below the buttocks.

MIDTHIGH: Stand on one foot, the other foot on a bench bent at 90 degrees, take the measurement on the thigh midway between the knee and the groin.

CALF: Stand erect, legs slightly apart (8 inches), take a horizontal measurement at the maximum circumference between the knee and ankle.

SET YOUR GOALS
THEN DEMOLISH THEM

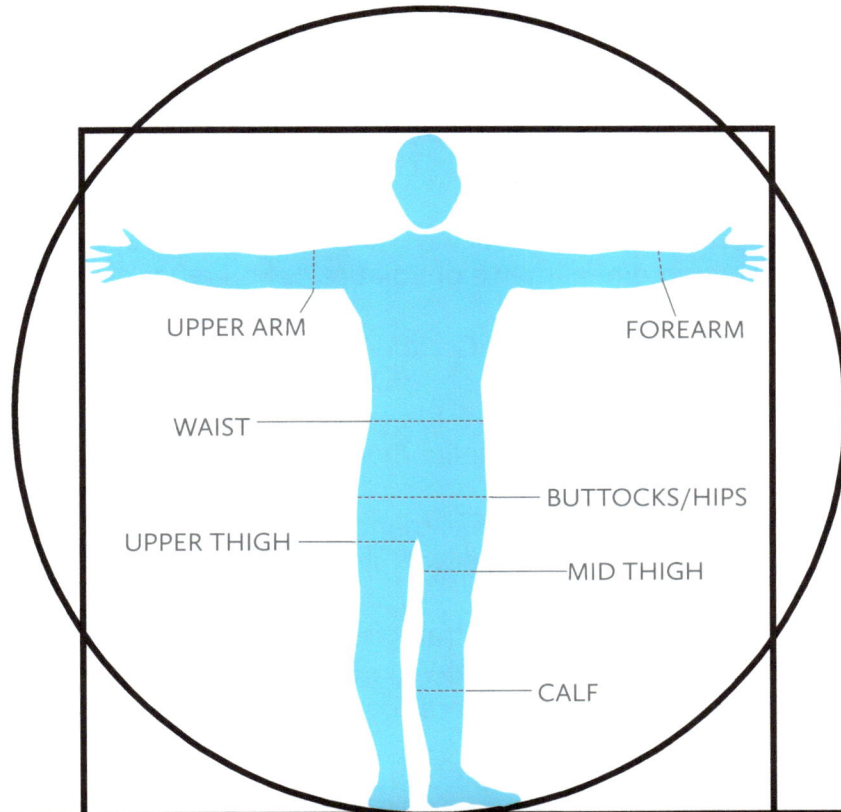

UPPER ARM
FOREARM
WAIST
BUTTOCKS/HIPS
UPPER THIGH
MID THIGH
CALF

MEASUREMENT	NOW	M1	M2	M3	GOAL
WEIGHT					
% BODY FAT					
UPPER ARM (R/L)					
FOREARM (R/L)					
WAIST					
BUTTOCKS / HIPS					
UPPER THIGH (R/L)					
MID THIGH (R/L)					
CALF (R/L)					

REFERENCES

Anne Bucher. "Atkins Class Action Lawsuit Says 'Net Carbs' Claims Are Deceptive." Top Class Actions, 19 Aug. 2017, topclassactions.com/lawsuit-settlements/lawsuit-news/813836-atkins-class-action-lawsuit-says-net-carbs-claims-deceptive/.

"Diet Review: Ketogenic Diet for Weight Loss." The Nutrition Source, 7 May 2018, www.hsph.harvard.edu/nutritionsource/healthy-weight/diet-reviews/ketogenic-diet/.

"Guidance for Industry: The Declaration of Certain Isolated or Synthetic Non-Digestible Carbohydrates as Dietary Fiber on Nutrition and Supplement Facts Labels" Accessdata.fda.gov, https://www.fda.gov/Food/GuidanceRegulation/GuidanceDocumentsRegulatoryInformation/ucm610111.htm.

"Food Labeling" Accessdata.fda.gov, U.S. Food and Drug Administration, 14 Sep. 2018, https://www.accessdata.fda.gov/scripts/InteractiveNutritionFactsLabel/dietary-fiber.html

Gibson, Alice A., and Amanda Sainsbury. "Strategies to Improve Adherence to Dietary Weight Loss Interventions in Research and Real-World Settings." Behavioral Sciences, MDPI, Sept. 2017, www.ncbi.nlm.nih.gov/pmc/articles/PMC5618052/.

Hemingway C, Freeman JM, Pillas DJ, and Pyzik PL. "The Ketogenic Diet: a 3- to 6-Year Follow-up of 150 Children Enrolled Prospectively." Pediatrics, U.S. National Library of Medicine, Oct. 2001, www.ncbi.nlm.nih.gov/pubmed/11581442/.

Lattimer, James M., and Mark D. Haub. "Effects of Dietary Fiber and Its Components on Metabolic Health." Nutrients, MDPI, Dec. 2010, www.ncbi.nlm.nih.gov/pmc/articles/PMC3257631/.

Likhodii SS, Musa K, and Cunnane SC. "Breath Acetone as a Measure of Systemic Ketosis Assessed in a Rat Model of the Ketogenic Diet." Clinical Chemistry., U.S. National Library of Medicine, Jan. 2002, www.ncbi.nlm.nih.gov/pubmed/11751546.

Musa-Veloso K, Likhodii SS, and Cunnane SC. "Breath Acetone Is a Reliable Indicator of Ketosis in Adults Consuming Ketogenic Meals." The American Journal of Clinical Nutrition., U.S. National Library of Medicine, July 2002, www.ncbi.nlm.nih.gov/pubmed/12081817.

"National Center for Health Statistics." Centers for Disease Control and Prevention, Centers for Disease Control and Prevention, 3 May 2017, www.cdc.gov/nchs/fastats/obesity-overweight.htm.

Neal, Elizabeth. "Dietary Treatment of Epilepsy: Practical Implementation of Ketogenic Therapy." Wiley-Blackwell, 2012. Pendick, Daniel. "How Much Protein Do You Need Every Day?" Harvard Health Blog, 8 Jan. 2018, www.health.harvard.edu/blog/how-much-protein-do-you-need-every-day-201506188096.

Pendick, Daniel. "How Much Protein Do You Need Every Day?" Harvard Health Blog, 8 Jan. 2018, www.health.harvard.edu/blog/how-much-protein-do-you-need-every-day-201506188096.

Shifflett, Tammy, et al. "Diabetes & Ketogenic Diet: Managing Diabetes On A Ketogenic Diet." TheDiabetesCouncil.com, 28 Sept. 2018, www.thediabetescouncil.com/can-you-manage-your-diabetes-on-a-ketogenic-diet/.

Spaněl P, Dryahina K, Rejšková A, Chippendale TW, and Smith D. "Breath Acetone Concentration; Biological Variability and the Influence of Diet." Physiological Measurement., U.S. National Library of Medicine, Aug. 2011, www.ncbi.nlm.nih.gov/pubmed/21725144.

"Sugar Alcohols." American Diabetes Association, www.diabetes.org/food-and-fitness/food/what-can-i-eat/understanding-carbohydrates/sugar-alcohols.html.

"Taking a Closer Look At Labels." American Diabetes Association, www.diabetes.org/food-and-fitness/food/what-can-i-eat/food-tips/taking-a-closer-look-at-labels.html.

Turton, Jessica L., et al. "Low-Carbohydrate Diets for Type 1 Diabetes Mellitus: A Systematic Review." PLOS ONE, Public Library of Science, 29 Mar. 2018, journals.plos.org/plosone/article?id=10.1371%2Fjournal.pone.0194987.

Wheeler, Madelyn. "What Are Net Carbs?" Diabetes Forecast, Aug. 2010, http://www.diabetesforecast.org/2010/aug/what-are-net-carbs.html.

NOTES

NOTES

NOTES

NOTES

NOTES

NOTES

RESOURCES

DRAEKK

draekk.com Your source for Performance Development, Time Management, and Keto Fueled Weight Loss. The company that brought you the CONCEPT24® Planner and the KT Diet. Visit the website for additional resources on keto recipes, exercises, and time management tips.

USDA FOOD COMPOSITION DATABASE

ndb.nal.usda.gov/ndb/search/list The USDA Food Composition Database is a great and accurate resource to get your nutritional information.

INDEX

RECIPE INDEX

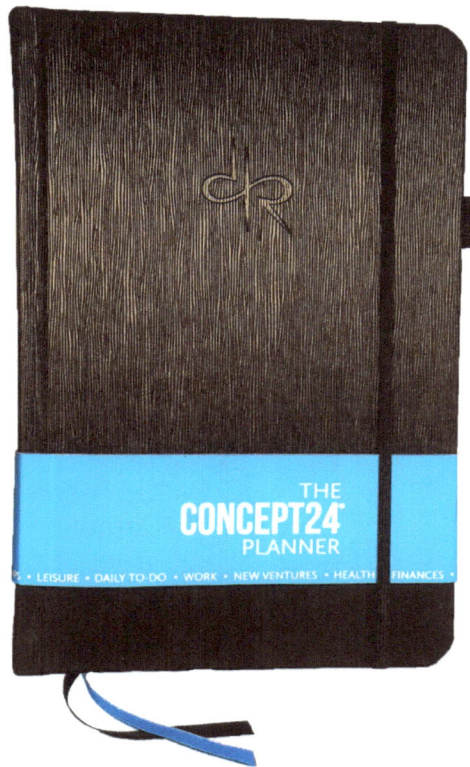

www.ingramcontent.com/pod-product-compliance
Lightning Source LLC
Chambersburg PA
CBHW060811270326
41928CB00003B/54